HEALTH CARE ISSUES, COSTS AND ACCESS

TRANSFORMING HEALTHCARE WITH HEALTH INFORMATION TECHNOLOGY

HEALTH CARE ISSUES, COSTS AND ACCESS

Additional books in this series can be found on Nova's website under the Series tab.

Additional E-books in this series can be found on Nova's website under the E-books tab.

HEALTH CARE ISSUES, COSTS AND ACCESS

TRANSFORMING HEALTHCARE WITH HEALTH INFORMATION TECHNOLOGY

CHARLES M. DENISON
AND
ELIZABETH L. MONTEVOY
EDITORS

Nova Science Publishers, Inc.
New York

Library of Congress Cataloging-in-Publication Data

Transforming healthcare with health information technology / editors, Charles M. Denison and Elizabeth L. Montevoy.
p. cm.
Includes bibliographical references and index.
ISBN 978-1-61324-417-3 (hardcover)
1. Medical informatics--Law and legislation--United States. 2. Data protection--Law and legislation--United States. 3. United States. Health Information Technology for Economic and Clinical Health Act. I. Denison, Charles M. II. Montevoy, Elizabeth L.
[DNLM: 1. Delivery of Health Care--legislation & jurisprudence--United States. 2. Medical Informatics--legislation & jurisprudence--United States. W 32.5 AA1]
K3611.R43A2 2011
344.7303'21--dc23

2011013416

Published by Nova Science Publishers, Inc. † New York

CONTENTS

PREFACE

Information technology (IT) has the potential to transform healthcare as it has transformed many parts of our economy and society in recent decades. Despite this great promise, the impact of IT on healthcare over the past decade has so far been modest. Compared to other industrialized nations, the United States lags far behind in the use of electronic health records. This book examines how health information technology could improve the quality of healthcare and reduce its cost, and whether existing Federal efforts in health information technology are optimized for these goals.

Chapter 1- Information technology (IT) has the potential to transform healthcare as it has transformed many parts of our economy and society in recent decades. Properly implemented, health IT can:

- Integrate technology into the flow of clinical practice as an asset, while minimizing unproductive data entry work.
- Give clinicians real-time access to complete patient data, and provide them with information support to make the best decisions.
- Help patients become more involved in their own care.
- Enable a range of population-level public health monitoring and real-time research.
- Improve clinical trials, leading to more rapid advances in personalized medicine.
- Streamline processes, increase their transparency, and reduce administrative overhead, as it has in other industries.
- Lead to the creation of new high-technology markets and jobs.
- Help support a range of economic reforms in the healthcare system that will be needed to address our Nation's long-term fiscal challenges.

Chapter 2- Lawmakers incorporated the Health Information Technology for Economic and Clinical Health (HITECH) Act as part of the American Recovery and Reinvestment Act of 2009 (H.R. 1), the economic stimulus bill that the President signed into law on February 17, 2009 (P.L. 111-5). The HITECH Act is intended to promote the widespread adoption of health information technology (HIT) to support the electronic sharing of clinical data among hospitals, physicians, and other health care stakeholders. HIT is widely viewed as a necessary and vital component of health care reform. It encompasses interoperable electronic health records (EHRs)—including computerized systems to order tests and medications, and support systems to aid clinical decision making—and the development of a national health information network to permit the secure exchange of electronic health information among providers.

Chapter 3- President Obama signed the American Recovery and Reinvestment Act of 2009 (P.L. 111-5) on February 17, 2009. Title XIII of Division A and Title IV of Division B of that act are referred to as the Health Information Technology for Economic and Clinical Health Act (HITECH Act). The HITECH Act was designed to promote the widespread adoption of health information technology (HIT). HIT involves the exchange of health information in an electronic environment.

Chapter 4- Electronic health information exchange promises an array of potential benefits for individuals and the U.S. health care system through improved clinical care and reduced cost. At the same time, this environment also poses new challenges and opportunities for protecting individually identifiable health information. In health care, accurate and complete information about individuals is critical to providing high quality, coordinated care. If individuals and other participants in a network lack trust in electronic exchange of information due to perceived or actual risks to individually identifiable health information or the accuracy and completeness of such information, it may affect their willingness to disclose necessary health information and could have life-threatening consequences. A key factor to achieving a high-level of trust among individuals, health care providers, and other health care organizations participating in electronic health information exchange is the development of, and adherence to, a consistent and coordinated approach to privacy and security. Clear, understandable, uniform principles are a first step in developing a consistent and coordinated approach to privacy and security and a key component to building the trust required to realize the potential benefits of electronic health information exchange.

In: Transforming Healthcare with Health Information…
Editors: C. M. Denison, E. L. Montevoy
ISBN: 978-1-61324-417-3

Chapter 1

REALIZING THE FULL POTENTIAL OF HEALTH INFORMATION TECHNOLOGY TO IMPROVE HEALTHCARE FOR AMERICANS: THE PATH FORWARD*

Executive Office of the President
President's Council of Advisors on Science and Technology

ABOUT THE PRESIDENT'S COUNCIL OF ADVISORS ON SCIENCE AND TECHNOLOGY

The President's Council of Advisors on Science and Technology (PCAST) is an advisory group of the nation's leading scientists and engineers, appointed by the President to augment the science and technology advice available to him from inside the White House and from cabinet departments and other Federal agencies. PCAST is consulted about and often makes policy recommendations concerning the full range of issues where understandings from the domains of science, technology, and innovation bear potentially on the policy choices before the President. PCAST is administered by the White House Office of Science and Technology Policy (OSTP).

For more information about PCAST, see
http://www.whitehouse.gov/ostp/pcast

* This is an edited, reformatted and augmented version of a President's Council of Advisors on Science and Technology publication, dated December 2010.

The President's Council of Advisors on Science and Technology

Co-Chairs

John P. Holdren
Assistant to the President
for Science and Technology
Director, Office of Science and
Technology Policy

Eric Lander
President, Broad Institute of
Harvard and MIT

Harold Varmus[1]
President, Memorial Sloan-Kettering Cancer Center

Members

Rosina Bierbaum
Dean, School of Natural Resources and
Environment
University of Michigan

Christine Cassel
President and CEO, American Board of Internal Medicine

Christopher Chyba
Professor, Astrophysical Sciences and International Affairs
Director, Program on Science and Global SecurityPrinceton University

S. James Gates, Jr.
John S. Toll Professor of Physics
Director, Center for String and Particle Theory
University of Maryland

Shirley Ann Jackson
President,
Rensselaer Polytechnic Institute

[1] Dr. Varmus resigned from PCAST on July 9, 2010 and subsequently became Director of the National Cancer Institute (NCI).

Richard C. Levin
President
Yale University

Chad Mirkin
Rathmann Professor, Chemistry, Materials
Science and Engineering, Chemical and
Biological Engineering and Medicine
Director, International Institute of
NanotechnologyNorthwestern University

Mario Molina
Professor, Chemistry and Biochemistry
University of California, San Diego
Professor, Center for Atmospheric Sciences
Scripps Institution of Oceanography
Director, Mario Molina Center for Energy and
Environment, Mexico City

Ernest J. Moniz
Cecil and Ida Green Professor of Physics and
Engineering Systems
Director, MIT's Energy Initiative
Massachusetts Institute of Technology

Craig Mundie
Chief Research and Strategy Officer
Microsoft Corporation

Ed Penhoet
Director, Alta Partners
Professor Emeritus of Biochemistry
and of Public Health
University of California, Berkeley

William Press
Raymer Professor in Computer Science and
Integrative Biology
University of Texas at Austin

Maxine Savitz
Vice President
National Academy of Engineering

Barbara Schaal
Chilton Professor of Biology
Washington University
Vice President, National Academy of Sciences

Eric Schmidt
Chairman and CEO
Google, Inc.

Daniel Schrag
Sturgis Hooper Professor of Geology
Professor, Environmental Science and Engineering
Director, Harvard Universitywide Center for Environment
Harvard University

David E. Shaw
Chief Scientist, D.E. Shaw Research
Senior Research Fellow, Center for Computational Biology and Bioinformatics
Columbia University

Ahmed Zewail
Linus Pauling Professor of Chemistry and Physics
Director, Physical Biology Center
California Institute of Technology

Staff

Deborah Stine
Executive Director, PCAST

Mary Maxon
Deputy Executive Director, PCAST

Gera Jochum
Policy Analyst

Executive Office of the President
President's Council of Advisors on Science and Technology
Washington, D.C. 20502

President Barack Obama
The White House
Washington, DC 20502
Dear Mr. President,

We are pleased to send you this report, *Realizing the Full Potential of Health Information Technology to Improve Healthcare for Americans: The Path Forward*, prepared by your President's Council of Advisors on Science and Technology (PCAST). This report examines how health information technology could improve the quality of healthcare and reduce its cost, and whether existing Federal efforts in health information technology are optimized for these goals.

To provide a solid scientific and economic basis for our recommendations, the Council assembled a Working Group of nongovernmental experts and also met with government officials, industry representatives, information technology experts, and healthcare professionals. PCAST has concluded that information technology can help catalyze a number of important benefits including improved access to patient data, which can help clinicians as they diagnose and treat patients and patients themselves as they strive to take more control over their health; streamlined monitoring of public health patterns and trends; an enhanced ability to conduct clinical trials of new diagnostic methods and treatments; and the creation of new high-technology markets and jobs. Health information technology can also help support a range of healthcare-related economic reforms needed to address our Nation's long-term fiscal challenges.

PCAST has also concluded that to achieve these objectives it is crucial that the Federal Government facilitate the nationwide adoption of a universal exchange language for healthcare information and a digital infrastructure for locating patient records while strictly ensuring patient privacy. More specifically, PCAST recommends that the Office of the National Coordinator for Health Information Technology and the Centers for Medicare and Medicaid Services develop guidelines to spur adoption of such a language and to facilitate a transition from traditional electronic health records to the use of healthcare data tagged with privacy and security specifications.

PCAST hopes that its report will help lay a foundation for the decisions that you and others in the Federal Government must make. We are grateful for the opportunity to serve you and the country in this way and would be pleased to brief you or your staff if you have questions about our recommendations.

Sincerely,

John P. Holdren, Co-Chair
Eric Lander, Co-Chair

Executive Summary

Information technology (IT) has the potential to transform healthcare as it has transformed many parts of our economy and society in recent decades. Properly implemented, health IT can:

- Integrate technology into the flow of clinical practice as an asset, while minimizing unproductive data entry work.
- Give clinicians real-time access to complete patient data, and provide them with information support to make the best decisions.
- Help patients become more involved in their own care.
- Enable a range of population-level public health monitoring and real-time research.
- Improve clinical trials, leading to more rapid advances in personalized medicine.
- Streamline processes, increase their transparency, and reduce administrative overhead, as it has in other industries.
- Lead to the creation of new high-technology markets and jobs.
- Help support a range of economic reforms in the healthcare system that will be needed to address our Nation's long-term fiscal challenges.

Despite this great promise, the impact of IT on healthcare over the past decade has so far been modest. Currently, almost 80 percent of physicians—the majority in small, independent practices—lack even rudimentary digital records. Where electronic records do exist, they are typically limited in functionality and poor in interoperability. As a result, the ability to integrate electronic health information about a patient and exchange it among clinical providers remains the exception rather than the rule. Compared to other industrialized nations, the United States lags far behind in the use of electronic health records.

As we will describe, the Administration and the Congress have recently made major investments to ensure that Americans soon enjoy the benefits of electronic health records. The Administration has been moving rapidly to promote the adoption by physicians and hospitals of electronic health systems, including through recent, important rule-making for 2011. The President's Council of Advisors on Science and Technology has undertaken this report to examine the critical issues for the next phase, which has just begun, and to make specific recommendations to the Administration to ensure that the full promise of health IT is realized.

In other sectors in which IT has had a transforming effect, rapid progress has been catalyzed by wise technology choices that open up markets to competition and innovation. Such technology choices include the standardization of simple universal methods for the exchange of information across multiple platforms and organizations. In other sectors, universal exchange standards have resulted in new products that knit together fragmented systems into a unified infrastructure. The resulting "network effect"[1] then increases the value of the infrastructure for all, and spurs rapid adoption. By contrast, health IT has not made this transition. The market for new products and services based on health IT remains relatively small and undeveloped compared with corresponding markets in most other sectors of the economy, and there is little or no network effect to spur adoption.

Several identifiable barriers in the healthcare system currently discourage innovation and vigorous competition in the market to create effective health IT systems. First, most current health IT systems are proprietary applications that are not easily adopted into the workflow of a clinician's day, and whose proprietary data formats are not directly exchangeable from one system to another. It is difficult for data to be disaggregated, indexed, searched, and assembled to provide accurate information to treat a patient, because the context for individual entries in a record is often implicit at best. Second, most healthcare organizations that utilize electronic health records (EHRs) view them as purely internal resources, and have little incentive for investment in secondary or external uses, such as making them accessible in appropriate form to patients, to a patient's healthcare providers at other organizations, and in de-identified or aggregated form to public health agencies and researchers. Third, legitimate patient concerns about privacy and security make patients uneasy about participating in health IT systems or granting consent for their information to be used in research. Fourth, health IT has historically been oriented toward administrative functions, not better care. This is in part because, under the current fee-for-service payment model, the economic benefits of investing in health IT can rarely be realized by the provider or organization that makes the investment.

Some healthcare organizations have overcome at least some of these barriers and successfully adopted electronic systems that measurably improve care within their own organization. Kaiser Permanente and the Veterans Health Administration are notable examples. Other leading hospitals and clinics also employ electronic record systems that allow them to consolidate patient health data generated within their organizations. However, even these successes, upon closer examination, highlight the limitations of current approaches. They are usually "one offs," designed for the particular organization, not for a wide range of other types of practices. They are generally closed, and not designed for the exchange of data with a heterogeneous and geographically diverse set of other organizations that may serve the patient now or in the future. They typically require capital investments that are beyond the reach of most small clinical practices. And, they are too limited in scope, and few in number, to drive a vigorous market in technological innovation.

Recent Federal legislation has charted a new path forward. The Health Information Technology for Economic and Clinical Health (HITECH) Act, a part of the American Recovery and Reinvestment Act (ARRA) of 2009, authorized expenditures of at least $20 billion to promote the adoption and use of EHR technologies that would ideally be connected through a national health information network. Hospitals and physicians who make "meaningful use" of interoperable EHRs can qualify for extra payments through Medicare and Medicaid.

Responsibility for developing policies that implement the overall HITECH Act lies primarily with the Office of the National Coordinator for Health Information Technology (ONC). In this role, ONC works closely with the Center for Medicare and Medicaid Services (CMS), which is responsible for promulgating policies that relate to Medicare and Medicaid payment for meaningful use of EHRs under HITECH. ONC and CMS recently released final rules to implement the first phase of the HITECH Act, which begins in 2011. The ONC rule specifies the standards, implementation specifications and other criteria for EHR systems and technologies to be certified under HITECH and thus eligible for the Acts incentive programs while the CMS rule specifies how hospitals, physicians, and other eligible professionals must demonstrate their meaningful use of these technologies in order to receive Medicare and Medicaid payment incentives. Both sets of rules strongly indicate that standards and criteria for achieving meaningful use of EHRs will grow more rigorous in subsequent phases (2013 and 2015) as the technology continues to evolve and providers gain experience and sophistication in its use.

Given the national priority of health care reform, President Obama asked PCAST how health IT could improve the quality of healthcare and reduce its cost, and whether existing Federal efforts in health IT are optimized for these goals. In response, PCAST formed a working group consisting of PCAST members and prominent experts in both healthcare and information technology. Based on input from the working group, additional expert reviewers, and its own discussions, PCAST has reached six major conclusions.

1) HHS's vigorous efforts have laid a foundation for progress in the adoption of electonic health records, including through projects launched by ONC, and through the issuance of the 2011 "meaningful use" rules under HITECH. ONC has shown itself to be a technologically sophisticated agency, with outstanding outreach into the clinical community and good liaison with incumbent EHR system vendors. The Nationwide Health Information Network (NHIN) project has convened stakeholders and created an appropriate forum for the discussion of options. Strategic Health IT Advanced Research Projects (SHARP) in areas including network architectures and data use will produce important practical advances, as will work resulting from the establishment of a Federal "collaboratory" in clinical decision support. Importantly, the 2011 "meaningful use" rules recently released by ONC and CMS provide necessary first steps, and we endorse these rules.
2) In analyzing the path forward, we conclude that achievement of the President's goals requires significantly accelerated progress toward the robust exchange of health information. The initial approach to meaningful use has focused on driving physicians to adopt EHR systems that perform important quality-improving functions within the practice and, to a lesser extent, on developing capabilities for broader sharing. Though the rule expresses an intent to require more robust exchange of health information among providers at later stages of meaningful use, its initial requirements that EHR systems communicate with each other are very modest. This creates a danger that EHR adoption during early stages of meaningful use may exacerbate the problem of incompatible legacy systems. What is needed is a simultaneous focus on the capability for universal data exchange, able to unleash the power of the competitive market, to produce increasingly better and less expensive systems, and to create the "network effect" that spurs further adoption. While useful as an initial step, the adopted standards for data vocabulary and messaging will not be sufficient to advance the state of the art either of clinical practice or of a robust health IT infrastructure. Going forward, the critical issue is to facilitate progress by healthcare organizations by ensuring the creation and dissemination of a universal exchange language for healthcare information and an infrastructure for locating patient records, while rigorously protecting privacy and security. This would allow patient outcomes to become a larger part of meaningful use much more quickly, and make it less onerous for clinicians to generate and report a wide range of different kinds of information about the outcomes of their practice.
3) National decisions can and should be made soon to establish a "universal exchange language" that enables health IT data to be shared across institutions; and also to create the infrastructure that allows physicians and patients to assemble a patient's

data across institutional boundaries, subject to strong, persistent, privacy safeguards and consistent with applicable patient privacy preferences. Federal leadership is needed to create this infrastructure. While the ability to exchange and integrate health data offers great advantages to patients, the economic benefits of these capabilities do not accrue directly to specific providers, or to providers' incumbent EHR system vendor (if any). As a result, market forces are unlikely to generate appropriate incentives for the necessary coordination to occur spontaneously. The nature of this coordination as a public good requires Federal leadership in ensuring the creation of the capabilities. The development of EHRs themselves should of course be left to the private sector.

4) Creating the required capabilities is technically feasible, as demonstrated by technology frameworks with demonstrated success in other sectors of the economy. The best way to manage and store data for advanced data-analytical techniques is to break data down into the smallest individual pieces that make sense to exchange or aggregate. These individual pieces are called "tagged data elements," because each unit of data is accompanied by a mandatory "meta-data tag" that describes the attributes, provenance, and required security protections of the data. Universal exchange languages for metadata-tagged data, called "extensible markup languages" are widely and successfully used. Indeed, ONC's clinical document architecture standard (CDA) is such a markup language, and is an important step in the right direction. The indexing and retrieval of metadata-tagged data, across large numbers of geographically diverse locations, is an established, highly developed, technology—the basis of web search engines, for example. With ONC leadership, these technologies could rapidly be adapted and standardized for universal use in health IT. Innate, strong, privacy protection on all data, both at rest and in transit, with persistent patient-controlled privacy preferences, is likewise achievable, and must be designed in from the start.
5) ONC should move rapidly to ensure the development of these capabilities; and ONC and CMS should focus meaningful use guidelines for 2013 and 2015 on the more comprehensive ability to exchange healthcare information. ONC should act boldly to articulate a clear, common framework that will ensure that its various efforts converge into an effective healthcare IT ecosystem that serves patients and providers. The steps that must be taken can be accomplished within the required time frame. It can be accomplished via an *evolutionary* transition from traditional EHRs to a tagged data element model, along with a *more rapid* transition for the more limited purpose of data exchange by means of a universal exchange language. We note that these steps are not intended as an alternative to ONC's important work in promoting the adoption of electronic health records. Rather they are complementary to that work and will accelerate adoption.
6) Finally, as CMS leadership already understands, CMS will require major modernization and restructuring of its IT platforms and staff expertise to be able to engage in sophisticated exchange of health information and to drive major progress in health IT. This process has begun, but needs to be a more urgent priority for the Administration and Congress and should be funded as appropriate for an essential component of the Nation's healthcare quality and affordability agenda. A recently initiated National Research Council study of CMS's IT capabilities should result in

recommendations that will avoid replacing one inflexible architecture with another (a common trap in Federal IT acquisitions), but a successful outcome is at best several years away.

The approach that we describe requires that there be a common infrastructure for locating and assembling individual elements of a patient's records, via secure "data element access services" (DEAS). Importantly, this approach does not require any national database of healthcare records; the records themselves can remain in their original locations. Distinct DEAS could be operated by care delivery networks, by states or voluntary grouping of states, with possibly a national DEAS for use by Medicare providers. All DEAS will be interoperable and intercommunicating, so that a single authorized query can locate a patient's records, across multiple DEAS.

Advantages of Focusing on a Universal Exchange Language

Briefly, the approach described in this report, focused on the technical ability to exchange data in uniform ways, has multiple advantages:

- It will improve healthcare quality, by making it possible for a physician to integrate accurately all of a patient's medical information.
- It will improve healthcare quality and decrease costs, by making it possible for third-party innovators to compete to create widely applicable services and tools serving patients, providers, payers, public health officials, and researchers.
- It will provide much stronger privacy protection than available under current approaches, allowing persistent privacy assurances (including applicable patient preferences) to be attached to different kinds of information and using data-level encryption to prevent access of data by unauthorized persons.
- It will not require universal patient identifiers, nor will it require the creation of Federal databases of patients' health information.
- It will simplify the regulatory burden on providers, by decreasing the focus of meaningful use regulations on *ad hoc* list of data items.
- It will help U.S. industry leapfrog to the front of the pack internationally in health IT, by providing exchange standards that can be more broadly adopted by others.
- It will facilitate public health and medical research, by providing a secure way to de-identify data.
- It will not require that existing systems be replaced, but only be modestly upgraded or augmented by "middleware."

In short, the approach is designed to create robust ecosystem to support the needs of patients, providers, payer, researchers and the Nation.

Creating the ability for uniform exchange in an existing marketplace is a coordination problem; it is a public good that calls for Federal leadership in coordinating standards for health metadata and in creating economic incentives to adopt the standard. The definition of meaningful use and the rewards for being a meaningful user (and penalties for not being one) can be, if properly implemented, powerful mechanisms for doing this.

Finally, one must keep in mind that achieving the truly transformative effect of modern health IT infrastructure on the healthcare sector will also require that economic incentives are in place to improve the quality of care and reduce costs.

Recommendations

The final chapter of this report offers guidance to ONC and CMS and also makes an itemized set of specific recommendations. We urge ONC to augment its current "bottom-up" approach with a process that can generate "top-down" design choices that are carefully balanced between the goals of convergence and diversity. This is an appropriate government role and requires a more aggressive approach than has been taken in the early stages. We also discuss how ONC might, by standardizing a universal exchange language whose semantics is intrinsically extensible, unburden itself of a potentially never-ending and intrusive government role in the harmonization of health record meanings across all private sector products. An open, extensible language will allow products to compete, balanced with other competitive features, on the basis of the breadth of their abilities to understand multiple semantic realms. ONC's clinical document architecture standard (CDA) is an important step in the right direction, but needs more focus on data transmission, on innate privacy features, and on the enabling requirements of a more robust marketplace in new and innovative health IT products.

As regards CMS, we suggest specific ways in which the meaningful use process could be used to better advance more strategic national goals in health IT. Apropos of the much-needed overhaul of CMS's antiquated IT infrastructure, we emphasize the importance of not replacing one inflexible architecture with another and briefly suggest what a modernized, versatile infrastructure might look like. Fortunately, CMS now has new leadership, with the appointment of an administrator. A solid technical plan, with the necessary resources, will be now required for success.

Although ONC and CMS both lie organizationally within U.S. Health and Human Services (HHS), the dimensions of health IT are broadly consequential across multiple Federal departments, including Veterans Affairs (VA) and Department of Defense (DoD). Among our recommendations, we therefore suggest that the Chief Technology Officer of the United States in coordination with the Office of Management and Budget and HHS, develop within 12 months a set of metrics that measure progress toward an a operational, universal, national health IT infrastructure that has the desirable features that we have discussed. Focusing these metrics on operational progress, as distinct from research, prototype, and pilot efforts, will enable a more accurate continuing assessment of whether Federal efforts in health IT, including both executive initiatives and legislative mandates, are in fact supportive of the President's goal of increasing the quality, and decreasing the cost, of healthcare.

PCAST HEALTH INFORMATION TECHNOLOGY WORKING GROUP

Working Group members participated in the preparation of an initial draft of this report. They are not responsible for, nor necessarily endorse, the final version of this report as modified and approved by PCAST.

Co-Chairs

Christine Casse[#]
President and CEO
American Board of Internal Medicine

Craig Mundie[#]
Chief Research and Strategy Officer
Microsoft Corporation

Members

Peter B. Bach
Attending Physician and Full Member
Memorial Sloan-Kettering Cancer Center

Basit Chaudhry
Consultant, physician

Molly Joel Coye
Senior Advisor
Public Health Institute

John Halamka
Chief Information Officer
Beth Israel Deaconess Medical Center
Chief Information Officer
Harvard Medical School

Eric Lander[#]
President
Broad Institute of MIT and Harvard

[#] *PCAST member*
[#] *PCAST member*

Jonathan Levin
Professor of Economics
Stanford University

Louise Liang
Retired Senior Vice President
Quality and Clinical Systems Support
Kaiser Permanente

William Press[#]
Professor of Computer Science and
Integrative Biology
University of Texas at Austin

Stephanie L. Reel
Vice President and Chief Information
Officer
Johns Hopkins University and Johns
Hopkins Health System

Harold Varmus[#]
President
Memorial Sloan-Kettering Cancer Center

Staff

Mary Maxon
Deputy Executive Director, PCAST

I. INTRODUCTION AND OVERVIEW

Introduction

Improving the quality and decreasing the costs of healthcare are among the Nation's highest priorities. In 1960, healthcare expenditures represented about 5 percent of the United States' gross domestic product (GDP).[3] Today they represent about 16 percent—the largest share of GDP spent on healthcare among all major industrialized countries. Yet on critical measures of healthcare outcomes, such as life expectancy, infant mortality, and the number of physicians per capita, the United States ranks behind many other countries.[4] Our expenditures are not producing the results we should expect.

[#] PCAST member.

Information technology has the potential to transform healthcare as it has transformed many parts of our economy and society in recent decades. *Health information technology*[5] can allow clinicians to have real-time access to complete patient data, and provide them with support to make the best possible decisions.[6] It can help patients become more involved in their own care, which is especially important in managing chronic conditions like diabetes, asthma, or heart disease. It can enable a range of population-level monitoring and real-time research such as the detection of developing epidemics, health risks in the environment, or adverse events caused by medications. It can improve clinical trials, leading to more rapid advances in personalized medicine. It can streamline processes and reduce administrative overhead, as it has in other industries. It can lead to the creation of new, high-tech markets and jobs. Finally, it can help support a range of economic reforms in the healthcare system that will be needed to address our country's long-term fiscal challenges. As David Blumenthal, the National Coordinator for Health Information Technology, has written, "Information is the lifeblood of modern medicine, [and] health information technology is destined to be its circulatory system."[7]

Despite this great promise, however, the impact of IT on healthcare has so far been modest. Currently, almost 80 percent of physicians—the majority in small, independent practices—lack even rudimentary digital records.[8] Of those who do use electronic systems, most do not make full use of their potential functionality. The sharing of health information electronically remains the exception rather than the rule. The market for new products and services based on health IT remains relatively small and undeveloped compared with corresponding markets in most other sectors of the economy. While recent Federal initiatives have made some important advances toward changing this situation, healthcare has taken only the first few steps toward an electronic future.

THE ORIGINS OF THIS STUDY

Given the importance of healthcare to the Nation's future, the President asked his Council of Advisors on Science and Technology how health IT could improve the quality of healthcare and reduce its cost, and whether existing Federal efforts in health IT are optimized for these goals. In response, PCAST formed a working group consisting of PCAST members and prominent experts in both healthcare and information technology.[9]

The working group held meetings in Washington, D.C., on December 18, 2009, and in Irvine, California, on January 14-15, 2010, as well as additional meetings by teleconference. The viewpoints of researchers, policy analysts, and administrators from government, healthcare organizations, and universities were presented and discussed. Additional analysis of the current state of health IT implementation among the 80 percent of physicians who practice outside of large integrated healthcare organizations was performed by the Science and Technology Policy Institute (STPI).

A draft report developed by the working group was submitted to the Health and Life Sciences committee of PCAST. That committee submitted the draft to several outside reviewers, who made valuable suggestions for improvements. From the working group draft, the additional input, and its own discussions, the Health and Life Sciences committee produced the present report, which was discussed and endorsed (with some modifications) by the full PCAST in public session on July 16, 2010.

Analysis of the Problem

Several identifiable barriers in the healthcare system currently discourage innovation and vigorous competition in the market to create effective health IT systems.

First, the diffusion of IT within healthcare has been slow and oriented toward administrative functions. *Electronic health records* that contain patient information captured in clinical visits, through lab and imaging studies, and likely in the future from genetic tests, are a cornerstone of health information technology. Many healthcare providers, however, do not have the economic incentives and technical expertise to purchase and use EHRs. Physicians who do adopt EHRs often find they are spending extra hours each day to type in orders, notes from patient visits, or measures to be reported to CMS without receiving commensurate benefits. In addition, the fee-for-service payment model prevalent in U.S. healthcare does not create strong incentives to coordinate care, share information, or avoid unnecessary treatments, all of which are potential advantages of using EHR systems.

Second, the current structure of health IT systems makes it difficult to extract the full value of the data generated in the process of healthcare. Most electronic health records resemble digital renditions of paper records. This means that physicians can have trouble finding the information they need, and patients often wind up with poor access to their own health data and little ability to use it for their own purposes. Electronic records often do not include links to relevant information such as recent research findings or data on best practices that physicians and patients could use to make the best possible decisions. For reasons we discuss below, market innovation has not yet adequately addressed these challenges to the *usability* of electronic health records.

Third, standards and infrastructure are lacking that would allow information to be easily shared across organizations. Relevant information does not seamlessly move with patients who receive care from multiple providers. This leads to duplication and hinders coordination of care. The lack of data exchange also means that researchers and public health agencies have limited access to data that could be used to improve health systems and advance biomedical research. Present Federal initiatives, described below, have the effect of encouraging the development of local and regional *health information exchanges* (HIEs) that involve agreements to exchange data among clusters of organizations. These exchanges are hampered by the administrative burdens of developing agreements and by a lack of financial incentives to increase coordination and efficiency. It is also unclear how these exchanges might scale to a national level.

Fourth, patients are concerned that the storage of their health information in electronic form will make it easier for employers, insurers, government, or malicious electronic intruders to improperly access their records. This concern may make them unwilling to participate in health IT systems or grant consent for their information to be used in research, even though the aggregation of patient data to compare treatments and providers is a major benefit of health IT. Data can be *anonymized* by removing all personal identifiers from the data. But patients also may want to be re-contacted if analysis of their data reveals a problem with a medication they are taking or a treatment that could benefit them.

Some large healthcare organizations have overcome at least some of these barriers and successfully adopted EHR systems. The *VistA* system adopted by the Veterans Health Administration (VHA) has helped the Nation's largest integrated health system provide a highly regarded level of information technology supporting better care. Kaiser Permanente's HealthConnect system links all of Kaiser's nearly 9 million members to all of its more than 14,000 physicians and their hospitals, rehabilitation centers and long-term-care facilities, so that Kaiser physicians can retrieve data on any patient who has received services anywhere in its network. Other leading hospitals and clinics also employ electronic record systems that allow them to consolidate patient health data generated within their organization.

These successes, however, also illuminate the limitations mentioned above. Even the most sophisticated organizations generally do not have efficient means to exchange health information with other providers. When exchanges occur, they often take place through limited or pre-formatted messages, such as electronic prescription information, or through comprehensive patient care summary documents, which cannot easily be searched for timely information such as that needed in an emergency. In addition, the systems employed by these large organizations are engineered to meet the specific needs of the organization that owns them, so they do not provide an open and accessible platform for market innovation that might lead to improvements in usability or functionality.

The main objective of this report is to argue that if health information technology is to have a truly transformative effect, the Federal Government should push ambitiously toward a national health data infrastructure in which patient data are readily available to providers in real time, can be accessed in *de-identified* form by researchers and public health agencies, and in which a market for applications that enhance EHR usability and patient involvement can flourish, enabling a "network effect" that can spur further adoption. The report describes a technological approach that could lead to this vision being realized, while at the same time strongly protecting privacy (including, where applicable, respecting the persistent privacy preferences of patients), and also describes some of the accompanying economic and regulatory steps that are required.

The Present Federal Landscape

Recent Federal legislation offers a promising start toward these objectives. The Health Information Technology for Economic and Clinical Health Act, a part of the American Recovery and Reinvestment Act of 2009,[10] authorized expenditures on the order of $20 billion (with estimates ranging from $9 billion to $27 billion) to promote the adoption and use of EHR technologies connected through a national health information network. Under HITECH, hospitals and physicians who make "*meaningful use*" of interoperable EHRs can qualify for extra payments through Medicare and Medicaid.

Responsibility for developing policies that implement the overall *HITECH Act* lies primarily with the Office of the National Coordinator for Health Information Technology; however, ONC also works closely with the Center for Medicare and Medicaid Services which is responsible for promulgating policies that relate to Medicare and Medicaid payment for meaningful use of EHRs under HITECH. Both ONC and CMS recently released final rules to implement the first phase of the HITECH Act, which begins in 2011. The ONC rule specifies the standards, implementation specifications and other criteria for EHR systems and technologies to be certified under HITECH and thus eligible for the Act's incentive programs while the CMS rule specifies how hospitals, physicians, and other eligible professionals must demonstrate their meaningful use of these technologies in order to receive Medicare and Medicaid payment incentives.

Both sets of rules strongly indicate that standards and criteria for achieving meaningful use of EHRs will grow more rigorous in subsequent phases (2013 and 2015) as the technology continues to evolve and providers gain experience and sophistication in its use. For example, to qualify for meaningful use incentive payments in 2011, CMS will require providers to be able to electronically transmit medication orders, record patient information and problem lists, demonstrate use of decision support tools, test systems to exchange health information with other providers, and submit a small number of clinical quality measures; by 2015, CMS expects that to qualify for meaningful use of EHRs, providers will need to demonstrate greater use of decision support tools, higher levels of information exchange, and actual improvement in care coordination and patient outcomes.

The ONC also has moved to take a number of other useful actions in the short time since passage of *HITECH*. The ONC director and his staff have sparked needed awareness in the provider community, galvanized the experts and industry stakeholders, and created a momentum for change through open policy committee processes, several pilot frameworks, and the support of research in key areas. In addition, they have directly funded regionally based support systems for physicians and other providers, and supported several new programs and research initiatives designed to promote the use of health IT and the exchange of health information. ONC has distributed over $564 million to states and state- designated entities to enlist their leadership in facilitating health information exchange within their jurisdictions and across state lines. Moreover, ONC is sponsoring many demonstration projects that build useful momentum and develop valuable experience and buy-in. These have helped to create the prerequisite conditions where Federal leadership, leading to rapid progress, is now possible. Further discussion of ONC's initiatives and successes is in Chapter Three.

Despite this progress, a major finding of this report is that achieving the President's goals depends on accelerating and redirecting current Federal work laying the groundwork for health information exchange. While the 2011 rules are an appropriate initial step, the approach underlying these rules will not suffice to ensure that the various activities and experiments being supported by ONC will converge into an effective healthcare IT ecosystem that serves patients and providers. Going forward, the critical issue will be to ensure the creation, dissemination, and use of a universal exchange language for healthcare information that enables health IT data to be shared across institutions, along with network infrastructure that enables a patient's data to be located and accessed across institutional boundaries, subject to strong, persistent, privacy preferences[11]. *ONC should move rapidly to ensure the development of these capabilities; and ONC and CMS should focus meaningful use guidelines for 2013 and 2015 on the more comprehensive ability to exchange healthcare information.*

We also have an important concern about CMS. CMS is the largest recipient of electronic health information (including data quality measures and measure sets) from hospitals and providers documenting their use and the effects of health IT. *CMS will require major modernization and restructuring of its IT platforms and staff expertise to be able to engage in sophisticated exchange of health information and to drive major progress in health IT.* This should be a major priority for CMS's new leadership, and should be funded as appropriate for an essential component of the Nation's healthcare quality and affordability agenda. A recently initiated National Research Council study of CMS's IT capabilities should result in recommendations that will avoid replacing one inflexible architecture with another (a common trap in Federal IT acquisitions), but a successful outcome is at best several years away.

Several other agencies within HHS have potentially important roles in health IT. The Agency for Health Care Research and Quality (AHRQ) is a small but increasingly important research agency supporting health services and delivery system research. Approximately 80 percent of its FY 2009 budget of $372 million is invested in grants and contracts focused on improving healthcare.[12] The Food and Drug Administration (FDA), while not currently regulating EHRs, currently does receive voluntary reports of death and injury associated with EHR malfunctions. FDA officials have suggested possible future regulatory strategies that could include mandatory adverse event reporting, or even classifying EHRs as medical devices, which would make them subject to pre-market regulation.[13] Other agencies with operational experience, such as the Centers for Disease Control & Prevention (CDC), or individuals in the Commissioned Corps of U.S. Public Health Service, might have roles to play in the management or operation of a future national health IT infrastructure.

Structure of this Report

Chapter Two gives a more thorough description of the benefits that could be realized by developing electronic health records to their full potential and integrating health information technology more completely into the healthcare system. The main features of the *data-centric* approach that we recommend are introduced with an initial discussion of *metadata*-tagged data elements.

Chapter Three describes in more detail the current state of health information technology, starting with the historical adoption and use of electronic records, and emphasizing the barriers that have arisen. The discussion focuses on specific cases that yield "lessons learned," both positive and negative. Also discussed are the successes and challenges facing the two key agencies ONC and CMS. The chapter concludes with a list of technical and market-related criteria against which to test proposed solutions.

Chapter Four outlines a technological approach based on the use of tagged data elements that could achieve many, if not all, of the key objectives. This chapter is somewhat more technical, although its general argument should be understandable by all readers. The deficiencies of solutions that require standardized records, or which rely on *service-oriented architectures,* are also noted.

Chapter Five summarizes today's privacy framework and indicates the ways in which it is inadequate for the future. Technologies are discussed that can be combined to achieve best-practice security along with persistent privacy protections.

Chapter Six discusses economic and regulatory issues, in particular how to reconcile the "public good" aspects of a national health IT infrastructure with the need to create vibrant, competitive markets. This chapter describes some of the main steps that are needed to complement the technological approach described in Chapters Four and Five, and relates health IT initiatives to the broader economics of healthcare.

Chapter Seven outlines some of the research opportunities that will be enabled by future health IT, and what are the requirements on that infrastructure so that the maximum benefits of that research can be achieved.

Chapter Eight brings together this report's recommendations and guidance to key Federal agencies. We offer guidance of both a general and specific nature to ONC and CMS, and also suggest what a longer term roadmap should look like. Among our key recommendations is that the Chief Technology Officer of the United States should oversee the development of a set of metrics that measure progress toward a national health IT infrastructure that is operational and universal (as distinct from experimental and pilot programs).

This chapter's bottom line: Health information technology has the potential to improve the healthcare system in numerous ways. Yet Federal efforts are not optimized to achieve the President's goals of improving the quality of healthcare and reducing its cost. Challenges differ by agency, but they include the need for more focus on the convergence of plans and the modernization of existing Federal IT infrastructure.

II. The Potential of Health IT

Introduction

In this chapter, we describe some of the potential benefits that could be realized from developing EHRs to their full potential and integrating health information technology more completely into the healthcare system. The benefits we describe might accrue at the level of individual clinical visits, at the level of healthcare organizations, at a broader regional and national level, and finally to patients wishing to have more information and more control over their own health and interactions with the healthcare system. We provide a series of "use cases" that illustrate the various levels at which information technology can improve healthcare delivery and the healthcare system.

We also note that formidable hurdles need to be overcome if these benefits are to be realized. The hurdles are both technological and economic. A key point is that current electronic health records, which are based on traditional paper records and exist largely within closed health organizations, cannot realize many of the potential benefits we have described. In order for health data to be broken down, indexed, transmitted across organizations, re-assembled, and aggregated, a more flexible technological approach is desirable. This approach is sketched below and described more fully in Chapter Four.

Later chapters expand on some of the other challenges that must be overcome to realize the potential benefits of health IT. Some early applications of IT in healthcare have had unexpected costs and consequences, and, despite the existence of commercial products and innovative demonstrations and pilot systems, the movement to electronic health records has been slow. The economic incentives to adopt and effectively utilize health IT have been weak, and the organizational structure of the healthcare system is itself highly fragmented. Current privacy regulation also creates complications for providers wishing to adopt and utilize IT. In short, there remain many barriers to achieving the potential of widespread and secure access to accurate, personalized, and comprehensive health data.

Potential Benefits of Health IT: An Overview

As medical practices and technologies have advanced, the delivery of sophisticated, high-quality medical care has come to require teams of healthcare providers, including primary care physicians, specialists, hospitalists, nurses, and technicians. Each member of the team tends to have specific but inevitably limited direct interactions with the patient. Every health provider has a somewhat different view of a patient, depending on the expertise the particular specialist brings to the medical team, and no one provider knows everything. In effect, the patient has fragmented into disconnected facts and clusters of symptoms. To prevent the most basic medical errors, some facts are elicited over and over again, to the frustration of patients and healthcare providers alike: "Do you have any drug allergies?" "Have you had any surgeries?" "Are you taking aspirin or blood thinners?" This frustrating repetition works, albeit inefficiently, if the patient is cognitively intact and well informed, but not all patients fit that description, especially in the event of a serious or acute illness.

Health providers need views of the patient that are less fragmented than at present. A cardiologist, for example, needs immediate access to a patient's most recent and significant cardiograms, cardiac imaging studies, and lab tests. He or she also needs to know about a family history of heart disease, concurrent illnesses being cared for by other specialists, past medical events, recent medications, and activity and nutrition changes. A nutritionist needs to know about a patient's serum cholesterol and also about life changes, such as a new job or the illness of a spouse, that may have caused a sudden change in the patient's diet. Health IT can integrate and organize patient information, and facilitate its instantaneous distribution among all participants in the healthcare system, so that providers and patients can obtain complete up-to-date views of each patient. In simple terms, health IT has the potential to put the patient back together again to allow more coordinated care.

Health IT also has the potential to generate valuable new information to improve workflow, safety, and efficiency within healthcare organizations. In industries such as manufacturing, retailing, and financial services, the efficiency gains from information technology were realized only when companies made complementary organizational changes. Today, some health organizations already use IT to track quality metrics, deploy reminder systems and checklists for physicians and other caretakers, and provide rapid feedback for the organization when changes are made. The widespread adoption of health information technology could allow these efforts to spread throughout the healthcare system.

The aggregation of data across organizations offers further possibilities. If the data gathered by healthcare providers and the decisions made at the point of care by providers and patients were gathered and aggregated, they could reveal patterns of illness in a community or nationally, identify potential epidemics at very early stages, enable comparisons of different treatments or medical devices in large and diverse populations, and evaluate the effectiveness of specific treatments and make information about hospitals, physicians, and other providers more comprehensive and accurate. Healthcare providers could use the information generated from these data to provide up-to-date and accurate guidance for patients, while healthcare recipients could draw on the data to prevent illness and obtain the best possible treatments. Data used to be an incidental byproduct of healthcare. In the future, timely information derived from high-quality data should be at the center of efforts to analyze, understand, and improve the healthcare system.

The next sections expand on these potential benefits of health IT, in part through simple "use cases." Readers may, and probably should, find some of these cases rather easy or obvious. Indeed, what is surprising is that today they are generally not possible in most care delivery environments.

Table 1. The Potential Benefits of Health IT

The ability to capture, store, exchange, and analyze medical information in electronic form could improve U.S. healthcare in many ways.

- **Quality of care for individual patients**. Patients will receive better medical care if they and their healthcare providers have access to complete and accurate electronic health records that aggregate information across time and organizations. Given the fragmented nature of the U.S. healthcare system, such integrated health records are now often not available. Such records could improve diagnoses, prevent errors, and save time.
- **Engagement of patients in healthcare**. The participation of patients in their own healthcare could substantially improve their care, especially in the management and treatment of chronic conditions such as obesity and diabetes. Access to electronic personal health information and interfaces that make it easy for public and private clinical organizations to share health information with each other and with patients could enable healthcare providers and patients to collaborate in informed decision-making.
- **Clinical studies of medical interventions**. Sound medicine needs to be based on empirical evidence of how well particular interventions work for patients. While some questions can only be answered through **randomized clinical trials**, a tremendous amount could be learned through the ability to integrate the combined experience of millions of patients. Aggregated de-identified information could enable a wide range of studies on such topics as the efficacy of prevention strategies, the frequency of particular complications in particular settings, and the response of individuals to specific drugs as a function of **genotype**.
- **Improved population-based knowledge.** Aggregated health information can provide invaluable tools for identifying and tracking medical events such as epidemics and adverse events related to treatment.
- **Development of new tools for medicine**. In most industries (such as retail consumer goods, shipping, and financial services), the availability of electronic information has led to an outpouring of creative tools that have increased quality and enabled new kinds of services. Healthcare could benefit greatly from such tools. Examples include home-based monitoring devices that could directly transmit data to physicians, systems that could help increase patient compliance with drug regimens, and computerized decision support systems able to incorporate the most up-to-date clinical knowledge.
- **Increased administrative efficiency**. In most industries, electronic information also has led to a decrease in administrative costs as many processes became automated. In healthcare, administrative tasks (such as filling out forms and processing billing requests) represent a significant fraction of healthcare costs. Health IT could streamline these tasks and significantly decrease costs.

The Value of Patient-Specific Data to Patients

Electronic health information should enable patients to have full and accurate information about all medical evaluations, to track the management of their own conditions, to schedule and change appointments as appropriate, and to exchange email with providers. This would give patients and families more direct engagement with their care, create an avenue for communication with healthcare providers, and identify treatable symptoms early to avoid unnecessary emergency room visits or hospitalizations.

> **Use Case 1:** A patient on warfarin, a blood thinner, strains his calf muscle during a tennis match and cannot remember whether it is safe to take Advil or Motrin. He types "Advil" into his personal health record list to see if there are any potential interactions with the list of medications in his record. Indeed, taking either Advil or Motrin would significantly increase his risk for serious bleeding. He emails his physician, who recommends cold packs and acetaminophen. The next day a discoloration and increased swelling occurs. He sends another email to the physician's office, where he is connected to a nurse practitioner who recommends a blood coagulation test. He is able to select times online for the test, for follow-up with the physician, and for possible further tests and physical therapy.

Electronic health information also can improve coordination of care by ensuring that every specialist, in every setting, has the same accurate and up-to-date information about a patient. This is especially important with patients who are seeing multiple specialists, with patients making transitions between care settings, and especially in emergency settings. This kind of data availability will reduce medical errors, reduce unnecessary tests, and reduce the chance that a patient's physician would not know about an unrelated but relevant condition being managed by another specialist.

> **Use Case 2:** A 70-year-old woman with a newly diagnosed lung mass suspicious for lung cancer discovered on a CAT scan in a small community hospital is referred to a large academic center in a metropolitan area two hours away. The patient's local hospital automatically makes available her electronic health record, enabling the cancer surgeon to pull up the CAT scan images and radiologist report at the patient's consultation. She doesn't remember all her medications, but her electronic record has recently been updated and verified. She may need a lung biopsy, and her record notes that she has an unusual cardiac arrhythmia that has been treated by a cardiologist in the past but that she is no longer taking medication. The biopsy is positive for lung cancer, and she will need both surgery and radiation. She is able to receive some of this treatment closer to one of her children, who lives in another state 1,200 miles away, with real-time communication electronically between her oncology team and her primary care physician. During this time, she is weakened and falls, sustaining a hip fracture. She is taken to the emergency room, where all her information is immediately available to sort out the otherwise confusing picture of cardiac arrhythmia, anemia from cancer treatment, and recent surgical scars.

The Value of Patient-Specific and Aggregated Data to Physicians

For the majority of U.S. physicians, electronic health information will for the first time enable them to query and analyze the "denominator" of their patient population—the full range of patients for whom they and their colleagues are responsible. This will make it possible for the physician to identify areas where patients are receiving less than optimal care—for example, how many patients with hypertension have their blood pressure under control, or how many patients with diabetes have their blood sugar measurements in the target range and have had appropriate screening tests.

This same clinical information is also essential to meet the growing number of demands for reporting of clinical quality measures for accountability and payment purposes. These demands are currently both expensive and cumbersome for most physicians, and to the degree that most of these data come from insurance companies, the data are limited to claims-linked information and are inevitably delayed and incomplete. Most physicians are very interested in and responsive to accurate evidence. Being able to interrogate one's own data for rates of performance on quality measures could lead to significant healthcare improvements.

Use Case 3: A general internist decides to seek approval for her practice to be designated a patient-centered medical home (PCMH) under Medicare because she cares for a large number of patients with chronic illness, including diabetes, heart disease, and hypertension. This requires her to submit a large number of data entry forms and quality measures, including descriptions of her patients, their disease profiles, and their demographics. Her office staff is able to do this easily by extracting the information from her EHR system, and she receives the designation. Her office is also able to file quality of care and utilization reports on a regular basis to 10 other payers apart from Medicare, and create reports that aggregate her patient population across all payers. This allows her to identify gaps in preventive measures or diabetes and hypertension control and create reports to maintain specialty board certification and hospital privileges. When she identifies areas for improvement, she implements changes in her practice and later re-measures. For example, she and her partners have increased the rate of elderly patients who received preventive falls assessments, and were able to do the follow-up measures electronically because they share EHR data with the two retirement homes and several nursing homes in the region. In doing this, they drew on patient-specific risk profiles and guidelines available electronically from the National Institutes of Health and the American Geriatric Society decision support programs.

Payers and consumers are increasingly including the results of patient surveys in performance measures used for payment, public reporting, and improvement. A fully functional electronic healthcare information system would enable physicians to contact patients directly, to solicit patient feedback related to specific conditions, and to compile actionable feedback to the practice.

> **Use Case 4:** A small group practice provides online access to each patient's medical record and communicates regularly with its patients via email. The practice has recently implemented an open access scheduling system and is curious to learn how patients feel about the change, so they email all patients with a recent office visit a web link to complete a focused satisfaction survey. They also participate in the Consumer Assessment of Healthcare Providers and Systems (CAHPS) survey authorized by Medicare but would like to add more specific questions related to patient's own conditions such as: "Did the nurse follow up with you about managing your new glucometer?" "Did your questions get answered?" They are able to personalize aspects of this survey and at the same time have only the needed aggregate data reported to payers.

As the use of quality measures increases, a question looms about how much real impact these measures will have on outcomes that are meaningful to patients. The combination of more efficient and accurate physician reporting with population-based outcome data could dramatically enhance critically important research about which of the measures link with desired patient outcomes, which of them lead most directly to improvement, and how to streamline the measurement and reporting process to reduce the time and financial burden on physician practices and still produce measures relevant to patient values.

> **Use Case 5:** A group of cardiology clinics in the Southwest, separated by significant distance, decides to work together to improve the care of patients who recently experienced a myocardial infarction (heart attack). They link information from each clinic's electronic medical records to track progress, learn what quality interventions work best, and create composite measures that help to distinguish what constitutes the best overall care. They are able to identify which sites have the best outcomes in certain areas, and they learn from each other how to apply these findings through webinars engaging all the staff in each clinic.

Having electronic health information about the entire population of patients served by a given practice or provider enables queries about groups of patients who suffer from a specific condition, are eligible for spec ific preventive measures, or are currently taking specific medications. Among other things, this population-based view enhances the ability of the practice to identify and work with patients to manage specific risk factors or combinations of risk factors. It also can detect patterns of potentially related adverse events and enable patients at risk to be quickly and correctly notified. For example, when a previously unidentified medication risk comes to light (as in the case of Vioxx), it is easy for the practice to identify all the patients taking that medication and to contact them immediately. If fully linked to the patient's personal health record, this function would also apply to over the counter medications. Similarly, when a needed vaccine (such as H1N1) is available, the practice can identify the patients at greatest risk and communicate with them efficiently. Outreach, patient education, and notification about particular risks are made possible by this kind of system.

> **Use Case 6:** A family physician embeds electronic reminders that alert her when the patient she is seeing during an office visit needs preventive care. Each fall, the clinic queries the electronic record to see which patients will need an influenza vaccine and to automatically generate a reminder email and/or text message sent to the patient. When an unusual pandemic strain appears, with different risk groups, the database can be queried to identify and communicate with those patients who are at highest risk.

The Value of Population Data for Research and Public Health

If real-time concurrent clinical data about every healthcare encounter were stored electronically, such data could be combined, without personal identifiers, from a regional or national population to allow enormous improvements in the ability to track public health issues and to develop prevention and amelioration strategies in a timely manner.

For example, natural epidemics such as H1N1 influenza are currently tracked through a combination of voluntary reporting by physicians and emergency rooms to various public health authorities and to the Centers for Disease Control and Prevention. Social networking and use of the Internet recently have been shown to add significantly to this capability.[14] But neither of these methods is impeccably accurate and truly comprehensive or able to pick up nuances of epidemics from current clinical data. A fully functional health information network that was widely used, interoperable, and able to be aggregated with a reasonable degree of accuracy and reliability would dramatically improve the ability to track known epidemics, to identify new ones, and to identify at an early stage other threats to public health such as bioterrorism or environmental exposures.

With sophisticated modeling expertise, this same database would enable *comparative effectiveness research* by tracking groups of patients taking comparable treatments for similar conditions. The results of these virtual clinical trials would be more representative of real-life patient populations, far less costly to conduct, and quicker to identify information relevant to the care of specific patient groups. Furthermore, as medicine is connected more closely to genetically linked traits and susceptibilities, this kind of tracking will accelerate the ability to provide patient-specific information to physicians and patients to individualize treatment decisions.

> **Use Case 7:** A physician treating a patient with rheumatoid arthritis using TNF (tumor necrosis factor) inhibitors enters the patient into the database of a national clinical study. Because the patient's clinical and genetic information are both known, the physician is able to use specific characteristics to predict outcomes and reduce toxicity without relying on the traditional trial and error process. This information is available to all physicians and patients and is continually updated.

This de-identified but clinically rich database would also enable *post-marketing surveillance* for FDA-approved medications, which now depend on voluntary reporting by physicians and healthcare organizations. An efficient way to track patient populations taking new medications, including other prescribed or over-the-counter medications simultaneously being administered, adds tremendous power to the ability to pick up adverse events or medication interactions as early as possible. As genetic information becomes more routinely available, this kind of post-marketing research capability will enable more accurate prescribing. This is especially important for medications such as biological (or cell-based) therapies and cancer chemotherapies where potential toxicities are significant and current research methods necessitate exposing large numbers of people to toxic side effects when they might not benefit from the treatment.

> **Use Case 8:** An FDA Commissioner is able to launch a real-time assessment of every patient taking newly approved drugs and aggregate clinical patterns to identify adverse side effects of medications. A robust post-marketing electronic registry allows much earlier detection of important adverse events for discrete subpopulations of patients and at negligible additional cost to FDA.

Population-based clinical data will enable communities, states, and regions to track their own health statistics in a more timely, reliable, and credible manner. As we consider the potential of setting health goals for communities as well as for the Nation, these data would provide a continuous measure against which all stakeholders (healthcare providers, community groups, consumer and workforce advocates, businesses, and government) could engage around setting targets and tracking progress. Congress has established a process to develop national priorities for improving healthcare in the United States, engaging all the relevant Federal agencies plus multi-stakeholder public-private collaborations.

> **Use Case 9:** For a particular year, ambitious new goals are set to improve health measures. Communities, regions, and states are able to provide comprehensive and accurate annual reports on each of these goals, identifying gaps where special focus is needed and key areas for focus in coming years. This process does not require extensive additional data gathering by state and local public health entities. Rather, it uses the flow of de-identified information generated by regular population health and healthcare activities.

Realizing the Potential of IT: A Data-Centric Approach

The use cases above only scratch the surface of what might be possible if market innovation in information technology were to take off. A number of barriers, however, stand in the way. First, current electronic health records largely employ proprietary formats that are not directly exchangeable from one system to another. Second, it is difficult for data to be disaggregated, searched, and indexed because the context (what we will refer to as the metadata) for individual entries in an EHR is often implicit at best.[15] Third, current EHRs generally exist institutionally within closed healthcare organizations or disconnected small practices rather than being accessible in appropriate form to patients, to other healthcare providers, and in de-identified or aggregated form to public health agencies and researchers. Strong economic incentives and regulatory initiatives are needed to overcome these obstacles. The new economic and regulatory programs launched by HITECH may not be sufficient.

In order to foreshadow later chapters of the report, it is useful to engage in a brief discussion of the EHR itself. A first point to convey is that in virtually all of our use cases, the "user" of the data does not need to be, and indeed should not be, scanning through the entire health record. Instead, the user needs to be looking at an application layer that accesses and presents a limited amount of information from a given health record or set of records. We refer to the ability of applications to access and utilize data relevant to a variety of specific tasks as a data-centric approach. Fortunately, data mining and presentation is something that computers, augmented by communications networks and distributed data storage, are very good at. Unfortunately, it is not something that current EHR systems are optimized for. Instead, many of them function as something closer to an electronic version of the paper record, and communication across systems is sorely lacking.

We will argue in this report that to achieve even the more modest goals set out in this chapter will require an infrastructure and a "universal exchange language" that allow data to be shared and communicated for different purposes among diverse EHRs and other applications. We also believe that there is a natural technological approach which will facilitate a move in this direction and which, over time, will also lead to beneficial changes in the way that EHRs are structured. This approach begins with the observation that the best way to manage and store data for advanced data-mining techniques is to break it down into the smallest individual pieces that make sense to exchange or aggregate. We will refer to these kinds of data as "*tagged data elements,"* because each unit of data is accompanied by a mandatory "*metadata tag*" that describes the attributes, provenance,[16] and required privacy protections of the data. Modern, networked computers are particularly good at indexing, finding, and retrieving data that are discrete and "close to the surface," even when the pieces are distributed widely over many computer systems and data-stores. So storing data in this fashion can create an environment in which clinicians can access a *patient-centric* record tailored for each medical encounter, and in which health organizations, researchers and public health agencies can aggregate data for a broad variety of uses.

We expand on these points in Chapter Four by arguing for an *evolutionary transition* from traditional EHRs to a tagged data-element model, *and a more rapid transition for the more limited purpose of data exchange*. In the model we will propose, data can easily be aggregated and de-identified, and data do not depend on a single provider or a single vendor for use. The entities needed to facilitate this type of information-rich environment could be viewed as part of the national health infrastructure, like hospitals and clinical laboratories, regulated, but typically not operated by government entities , allowing data to be drawn safely for uses in multiple arenas. Embracing this outcome is an important and essential step toward leveraging the true power of information technology to improve healthcare.

CONCLUSION

Information technology, along with associated managerial and organizational changes, has brought substantial productivity gains to manufacturing, retailing, and many other industries.[17] Healthcare is poised to make a similar transition, but some basic changes in approach are needed to realize the potential of healthcare IT.

The most significant change is that all healthcare should be organized around the needs and specific characteristics of the patient, not around those of the hospital, doctor's office, insurance company, or EHR vendor. Medicine has become an information-rich enterprise, and a larger and more seamless flow of information will result in a transformation of care, organized around the patient, wherever he or she may be. The healthcare system will be driven by information and at the same time will generate information that can be used to improve healthcare. The potential for individualized care, higher quality, lower costs, and enhanced safety is immense.

The best way to give clinicians a unified, patient-centric record tailored for each medical encounter is to store, maintain, update, and exchange the data as small, distributed, metadata-tagged elements. The data element indexing and access services needed to facilitate this type of information-rich environment can be viewed as part of the national health infrastructure, like hospitals and clinical laboratories. Embracing and promoting this outcome is an essential step toward leveraging the true power of information technology to improve healthcare.

This chapter's bottom line: Improved health IT can directly affect, and improve, clinical encounters between doctor and patient, healthcare organizations, clinical research, and the monitoring of public health. For this to happen, we must be able to "disassemble" the information in electronic health records and then "reassemble" it in various ways.

III. Health IT Today

Introduction

Traditionally, electronic records and information technology have played a limited role in healthcare delivery. There are a number of reasons for this, both economic and technological. In this chapter, we describe some of the historical barriers to health IT adoption, and the current Federal initiatives that are beginning to change the health IT landscape. In doing this, we touch on some of the lessons that can be drawn from the experience of early IT adopters, predominantly large integrated healthcare organizations, as well as the historical and current state of EHR technology.

The final part of this chapter discusses nascent attempts to promote data sharing through local and regional health information exchanges. Data sharing and exchange through a national health IT infrastructure is essential to realize many of the potential benefits described in the current chapter. This requires the ability to access, assemble, and present data that are potentially being generated across a range of organizations. This capability is by and large lacking in the current environment. Moreover, current approaches to data exchange and aggregation, which are often bilateral or document-based, do not, in our view, present a clear path to scalable national solutions that would trigger transformative innovation and use of health IT. In this sense, there is potentially a large gap between the current path and the potential for IT to improve health and healthcare.

Historical Barriers to EHR Adoption

Although the promise of EHR systems was recognized decades ago,[18] even today the great majority of physicians rely on paper records and use electronic data mainly for billing purposes. According to the CDC's National Ambulatory Medical Care Survey (NAMCS, 2009) only 6.9 percent of physicians reported having an extensive, fully functional electronic record system. Only 20 percent reported having even a basic electronic record system.[19] At first glance, this is surprising given that computers and information technology are so completely embedded in most industries. One would be shocked to hear of a leading manufacturer using paper records to track production or inventories, or of a financial services firm relying primarily on faxes and ordinary mail to exchange information with clients and partner firms. Indeed, healthcare providers have long used computers and IT for billing and communication with payers. Why has the broader adoption and utilization of information technology in healthcare been so slow?

At least part of the explanation lies in the organizational and economic structure of healthcare. Most physicians practice in small groups and are reimbursed for care on a fee-for-service basis. Physicians operating in this type of environment cannot easily internalize many of the potential benefits of electronic records and health IT, such as improved sharing of patient information, greater coordination of care, and aggregation of data.[20] They also have little incentive to undertake the substantial investment or money and time to install and adapt to electronic records, particularly when this involves a large fixed cost that cannot be spread across a large number of patients or physicians.

The situation has been compounded by a number of additional factors. Lacking demand from providers, the market has been slow to provide IT products geared toward small organizations. As we discuss below, even the advanced systems geared toward hospitals and large healthcare providers lack capabilities that seem rather obvious, such as extensive clinical decision support, or the ability to easily exchange data with other providers who share responsibility for the same patients. In addition, privacy and liability concerns may be a deterrent for some organizations, or at least for data-sharing initiatives.

Not surprisingly, the healthcare organizations that have adopted electronic health records tend to be large organizations that can shoulder the financial burden of installing customized systems and can internalize the benefits associated with such systems. These systems also tend to have different financial incentives than are prevalent in the broader healthcare system. Some are paid on a capitated basis (a fixed amount per patient per year), so they have an incentive to provide care efficiently and reduce duplication or extraneous services when possible. However, some tens of thousands of small physician practices have also adopted electronic health records. These physician adopters tend to be younger and more technologically savvy than their peers. Below we discuss some of the lessons that can be gleaned from the experiences of these early adopters.

Limitations of Present-Day EHRs

The most commonly cited reasons for not adopting EHRs include the cost of installing and maintaining a system (including both financial and workflow disruption costs) and the lack of perceived benefits in terms of enabling higher quality, more efficient care. A frequent complaint is that electronic health records do not make the physician's job easier. In particular, few EHRs deliver the intelligent cognitive or decision support that one might hope for. Even where decision support is available, physicians often do not take advantage of it. This section describes some of the cost and "usability" concerns around current EHR systems, and how a robust technology market could alter the situation.

Workflow Disruption and Documentation Burden

Present-day EHRs often require a substantial increase in physician time devoted to documentation. Physicians may complain that they are spending extra hours to type in orders and notes from patient visits. Healthcare systems can hire staff to enter data into the EHR during the office visit, but this is cumbersome and not economically feasible for small practices. Speech-to-text transcription systems exist, but so far they are useful only for specialties with circumscribed and highly specific vocabularies. Physicians often are left to design their own "templates" to reduce the data entry burden. Streamlined data entry via checklists, customizable templates, and other structured means is an area of opportunity for software and systems designers.

Lack of Decision Support Functionality

Many EHRs were developed as electronic facsimiles of existing paper records. They were created largely without the assistance of experts in human factors and design and they do not fully leverage the ability of computers to retrieve and analyze data to provide useful guidance, safety checks, and decision support. There have been some useful advances in this area, such as modules that cross-check for drug interactions, provide warnings about allergies, or generate reminders for preventive services. Nevertheless, this is an area ripe for innovation. Recently, the National Research Council proposed a comprehensive research agenda for the development of new approaches to EHRs that would provide cognitive support for clinicians and draw on human factors engineering.[21] As just one example of the potential, research over the past decade has raised the possibility that diagnostic errors may be far more extensive than therapeutic errors. As much as 15 percent of all diagnoses may represent clinically significant errors.[22] Clinical decision support that could assist physicians in making effective diagnoses might represent a significant opportunity if it could be integrated with the electronic record.

Technology-Enabled Diagnoses

Imagine a patient with the history of hepatitis C who presents to a primary care physician complaining of an itchy rash. When the physician dictates or types the words "new rash" into the record, the record instantly reminds the physician that hepatitis C has associations with certain diseases, including a condition known as lichen planus that triggers an itchy rash. The decision support system can remember all of the associations between patient clues and medical diagnoses. It then becomes the job of the clinician to navigate the evidence and assess the situation with the richer information that is instantly available. In another example, imagine a veterinarian presenting with new symptoms. The decision support engine would immediately display diseases associated with veterinarian exposures. Such functionality is feasible today, but the burden and costs of deploying the record, and the use of "first generation" decision support by vendors, have hindered critical innovations needed to reduce diagnostic and therapeutic errors.

Lack of a Platform for Innovative Applications

Many healthcare systems use enterprise systems customized to fit the needs of the particular provider. Other organizations rely on idiosyncratic "legacy" systems that often were initially used primarily for billing or pharmacy refills. Neither type of system provides an open and robust platform for software developers to build applications to improve data entry processes, provide decision support, or other functionality. The fact that existing systems often use record formats based on messages and page formats also makes it harder to access, retrieve, and analyze individual data elements. In addition, existing systems typically are not interoperable, so that data cannot easily be shared or aggregated across organizations. Although we discuss below some new technologies that may improve this situation, these limitations stand in the way of innovation that could help to alleviate some of the usability problems described above.

Concerns about Security and Privacy

Finally, a major concern with healthcare information, as with financial and other highly sensitive personal data, involves security and privacy. The Privacy and Security Rules issued under the Health Insurance Portability and Accountability Act (HIPAA) of 1996 provided the first broadly applicable Federal protections for health information. These Rules, along with multiple state laws, create a complex network of laws and regulations that address patient privacy and consent for the use of identifiable personal health information. The resulting regulatory framework, in current implementations, imposes significant costs on healthcare providers. Moreover, although HIPAA has usefully raised awareness of the need to protect health information, the Rule has become obsolete in many ways given advances in technology. A recent Institute of Medicine (IOM) report concluded that the law needs to be fundamentally reconsidered to reflect new information technologies and to enhance personalization and the quality of care.[23] Chapter Five expands on this point and discusses how emerging capabilities in metadata, encryption, and identity systems enable promising new ways to protect Internet-based information that were not envisioned when HIPAA was passed.

Lessons from Early Adopters

The healthcare organizations that have adopted electronic health records are mainly large integrated health systems that can internalize the benefits of EHRs as well as fund the initial investment and ongoing maintenance. Although these organizations are not necessarily representative of the broader healthcare system, their experience provides some important lessons.

The Kaiser and VA Experience

Two of the Nation's largest healthcare systems—the Veterans Health Administration (VHA) medical system and Kaiser Permanente—were among the earliest adopters of integrated EHR systems.

The VHA's adoption of its VistA system is credited with playing a major role in enabling the Nation's largest integrated health system to provide a highly regarded level of information technology supporting better care.[24] For example, the use of electronic reminders and performance measurement to improve pneumonia vaccination rates probably saved the lives of 6,000 veterans with emphysema.[25] VHA's vaccination rate became the national benchmark as pneumonia hospitalizations were halved even while VHA's patient population doubled—all while reducing taxpayer costs by $40 million.[26] VistA also has enabled the VHA to reduce medication errors to a rate of 7 per million prescriptions written, well below the national average of 1 error in 20.[27] VistA has been made available in open source but lacks the flexibility of other commercial systems, so it is not widely adopted except by some safety net organizations. It currently does not connect easily with other systems or *with personal health records* (PHRs, discussed below). Nor is it strong at creating searchable databases that web-based models promise. A descendent of VistA, the Armed Forces Health Longitudinal Technology Application (AHLTA), contains medical records of nearly 10 million military service personnel and their families. However, VistA and AHLTA have diverged to the extent that they are no longer cross-compatible.

Kaiser Permanente's HealthConnect system is based on the Epic EHR, the most widely used of current vendors. Kaiser's implementation connects all 8.6 million Kaiser Permanente members, over nine states and the District of Columbia, to 14,000 physicians[28] in Kaiser's 431 medical offices and 36 hospitals.[29] Physicians can retrieve data on any patient who has received services within their network. Kaiser has used the system to improve preventive care and the management of chronic conditions. Specialists are alerted if a patient is overdue for preventive screening (such as mammography), and often the test can be scheduled for that same day. Kaiser's system also produces quality measures and feedback for physicians, medical centers, and hospitals,[30] and is able to aggregate population-level data to track adverse events and trends. It was the first to identify the link between Vioxx and increased risk of heart attack and to remove the drug from its formulary.[31] It can also track early cases, predicting epidemics, such as influenza, across its offices.

An additional feature of Kaiser's IT system is that it allows patients to access online data and communicate with their physicians using secure messaging. More than 3 million Kaiser patients are registered for this feature, and over 100,000 access the system on a given day.[32] Kaiser attributes this part of the system with improving both quality and efficiency of care delivery. Findings from a 2009 study showed that patients' use of secure messaging and scheduled phone "visits" enabled by HealthConnect led to a 26.2 percent decrease in total office visits over four years.[33] Over the same four years, most measures of healthcare effectiveness and patient satisfaction improved significantly. Despite this useful functionality, however, Kaiser's system is a closed one that does not communicate easily with other systems or networks. Only recently have Kaiser and the VA begun to collaborate to share data about patients who use both systems, and efforts so far are limited to one geographic area (San Diego). Kaiser also is exploring further interactions with health information exchanges in some regions.

Experiences at Other Organizations

The experiences of some other health systems help to illustrate the use of EHRs and the variety of issues involved in deploying IT in very different organizational and economic environments. In each of them, one can see the advantages to the patients within that system, but also the limits to models that are enterprise based rather than based on Internet technology.

The Palo Alto Medical Foundation (PAMF) is a highly-regarded multi-specialty group in Northern California that is affiliated with Sutter Health. In 1999, it deployed an Epic electronic record system similar to Kaiser's.[34] Physicians can pull up notes written by other PAMF physicians, access lab and imaging results, and send messages to patients. Physicians and administrators also have access to population-level quality measures. PAMF has used IT to alter the scheduling system so that many routine visits are scheduled just one or two days in advance. Because PAMF does not own its own hospitals and recently merged with two other large groups in the Sutter system, it has been attempting to make its systems compatible with its partners and integrate data fully across its component groups. Even today, however, it has not achieved full integration.

Geisinger Health System is a prominent health system in central Pennsylvania that encompasses both Geisinger's own health plan and affiliated clinicians. Geisinger has extended its EHR to include the private practice physicians in the community, allowing them to access information about their patients hospitalized at Geisinger Hospitals, and allowing hospital-based physicians to get access to records from the community practitioners. Geisinger maintains a corporate research center that aggregates data from all the providers in the system to produce clinically based measures of quality of care, help physicians establish benchmarks, and monitor quality for external reporting. The distributed aspect of Geisinger's system involves additional challenges such as the standardization of data elements and data systems that are integrated into central data repositories. It has been easier for Geisinger to do this because they it is essentially the sole hospital provider in a large geographic area, and it does not face the competitive forces that might deter community physicians from signing onto a EHR system that only provided information from one hospital system and not others where their patients might receive care.[35]

Lessons and Challenges

The experiences described above demonstrate how health IT can be successfully deployed and used, but they also reveal some of the challenges that remain.

A first point is that each of the organizations above has developed a system specifically tailored to its own needs. Each system has been expensive to deploy and requires substantial resources to maintain, as well as a significant and sustained effort to extract and utilize the information for organizational and care process improvements. While the organizations we have described also realize corresponding benefits, this kind of enterprise solution is inappropriate for small physician groups. Also, the patchwork nature of organizational solutions does not provide a scalable model for the effective flow of information centered around a patient, wherever that patient may be, or for a market for innovative electronic information solutions to everything from patient empowerment, to patient specific clinical decision support, to real time aggregated clinical data for robust quality assessment and public health purposes.

Second, the systems we have discussed are not mutually interoperable, meaning that patient information cannot easily be shared between providers with different systems or in different networks without a significant up-front investment to make this possible. Interoperability is important to improve and coordinate care delivery. Currently in the United States, most patients receive care from a variety of providers. One recent study found that the typical Medicare patient receives care from seven physicians spread across four organizations in a single year.[36] The lack of interoperability at the network level means that physicians do not easily have access to complete records for patients, nor does there exist a "master record" that is complete at any point in time. Chapter Six goes into more detail about the economic incentives for interoperability and how they can be better structured in the future.

Health Information Exchanges

Data exchange and aggregation are central to realizing the potential benefits of health IT. We have already seen the limitations of current systems in this regard. In this section, we describe some nascent efforts to create health information exchanges that allow for a degree of local and regional data sharing. We also discuss why these exchanges do not provide an obvious or immediate path toward a national health IT infrastructure.

Health Information Exchanges are entities often built on a series of often bilateral legal agreements between different, often proprietary information systems to be able to share certain kinds of data. Many HIEs were developed for the purpose of aggregating health measures at the community level, such as those supported by the Robert Wood Johnson Foundation (RWJF) in its Aligning Forces for Quality initiative.[37] Within this RWJF-funded group and in other instances, these HIEs have been termed regional health information organizations (RHIOs). Originally conceived in response to the fact that physicians, hospitals, insurers, and other healthcare entities have been reluctant to share data beyond their corporate boundaries, they are typically state or regional entities set up to facilitate health information exchange in a region or market area. Their primary responsibility historically has been to establish "trust relationships" among these entities in order to enable the broadest possible health data exchange. They also facilitate the governance, data-sharing agreements, scope, technology, and financial models needed to support that exchange.

Conceptually, HIEs might be considered the mirror image of the enterprise EHR model. Their purpose is to locate all currently available electronic information on a patient from any source, in that community or region, and present it in an integrated format to any physician who is authorized to view it. Current electronic sources for these data are national and regional laboratories, pharmacies, and clinical claims data. The physician sees, therefore, information from other physicians caring for their patient, records on medications, lab test results, and, as it is made available, copies of hospital discharge summaries and eligibility and claims status. However, HIEs have been limited by the administrative burdens of obtaining data-sharing agreements at every practice and every hospital or nursing home. They also have been hampered by a lack of financial incentives to develop more coordinated and efficient use of resources (including information resources), as described later in this chapter. In addition, the level of clinical detail in these contractual agreements does not match the richness of information available from a clinical record. Nevertheless, they do provide the treating physician with the information that generally is most important to know about a patient, which can make a very big difference in patient outcomes. As regards privacy and security, HIEs demonstrate the reluctance of providers to share data with users they do not know—generally, users outside the communities in which providers reside.

It is important to note that participation in an HIE does not require the physician to participate in any proprietary system or to invest in a fully functional EHR. The information summary for a patient can be presented through a browser or computer screen "dashboard" in the physician's office, faxed, or deposited into an EHR if the physician has one. Most HIEs provide a portal through which physicians can "plug into" an EHR to view information. While ultimately physicians would be expected to exchange, not simply view, patient health information, some have argued that HIEs provide an important "on ramp" for small practices and independent physicians and their staff to integrate the use of health IT into their practices prior to full EHR implementation.

Nevertheless, HIEs have drawbacks that make them ill-suited as the basis for a national health information architecture. One major concern is their durability. As a Federal strategy to support health information exchange, HIEs began in 2005-2007 with a small amount of Federal demonstration funding to states; a few also received private grant support. Barriers to their success were substantial, including complex governance, the lack of a sustainable business model, continuing provider reluctance to share data, the lack of readiness to accept and use data in many organizations and practices, and technical limitations in knitting together the many disparate IT systems within most medical communities. As a result, only a handful of the original HIEs have managed to establish exchanges that functioned beyond the initial funding and limited scope of their initial pilots. Recent legislative support for new state-designated HIEs and requirements for information exchange and reporting will clear away a few of these hurdles, but the lack of a clear business case for communities to sustain HIEs over time remains a daunting challenge.

Interoperability also remains a concern. HIEs are subject to differing regional and state-based governance frameworks. Also, limitations result from a lack of standards to connect multiple proprietary systems. There is no guarantee that a patient who has received care in two or three hospitals, has recuperated in a nursing home, and is now receiving home care and seeing several different specialists will necessarily have all her data available to a treating physician during an office visit or at an emergency event such as a fall and hip fracture.

New and Emerging Technologies

A number of new technologies offer significant potential for addressing the challenges described in the preceding sections. In this section, we describe three of them: cloud-based EHR products that are suitable for small providers, personal health records aimed at patients, and middleware products designed to make legacy systems interoperable. This discussion provides background for the next chapter of the report, which explains the technology issues associated with creating a health data platform that can facilitate innovation and broader transformation in healthcare.

"Cloud-Based" Technologies for Small Providers

As discussed above, the enterprise solutions used by early adopters are not obvious solutions for the smaller healthcare organizations that still make up a large fraction of the U.S. healthcare system. Small organizations need low-cost off-the-shelf products and services that can allow them to capture the benefits of health IT without having to undergo a costly customization and maintenance process. The incentives created by HITECH have already led to substantial innovation and competition in this area.

The new products often rely on *cloud-based* technology that allows software to be run and data to be stored on remote servers. The cloud model reduces individual maintenance responsibilities and allows even small organizations to benefit from the scale economies in data storage and processing. In this model, much of the responsibility for maintaining security is shifted from the small health care organization to the cloud-based service provider. It is also advantageous from the perspective of promoting data exchange because data from many organizations are stored and processed in a more uniform way. In the future, more extensive cloud-based solutions and services are likely to provide small or underresourced practices with everything from general practice management to advanced decision support to analytical tools for public health reporting and basic clinical research.

Personal Health Records

PHRs are patient-controlled repositories of individual health data. They may contain excerpts or summaries of physician records generated from clinical encounters, claims data, lab and imaging results, prescription information, and (importantly) patient-entered data. Some PHRs, such as those offered by Dossia, Google, and Microsoft are available via the web, while others are software packages that allow consumers to store and maintain data on personal computers, mobile phones, or other digital devices. PHRs can include functions such as decisions support, appointment making, referral requests, medication refills, and bill paying. Patients also can contribute their own data to the PHR and can determine what data will be accessible to clinicians and others.

To date, most PHRs are not standards based, and few support an easy way to transport records among different EHR products. However, Google and Microsoft, the two largest vendors of web-based PHRs, recently agreed on mechanisms to enable the free exchange of information between their respective PHR systems, and others may follow.

An important feature of PHRs is that they are patient controlled and "travel with" the patient. In this sense, they represent a route to interoperability. A patient could schedule a visit with a new physician, or a specialist, and allow access to his or her PHR. PHRs can also allow increased patient involvement in their own healthcare by enabling them to input their own data, research health issues, and potentially meet and share information with patients who have similar conditions. Of course, one question about this type of technology is how much interest patients will actually have in utilizing these capabilities. They seem to have particular promise for patients with chronic conditions.

Data Aggregation "Middleware"

An important feature of today's environment is that there is relatively little standardization in the health data captured and stored by different providers of healthcare services. Although a great deal of data already exist in the form of claims data, prescribing information, lab and imaging results, and clinical records, much of this data is trapped in different, incompatible databases. The last few years have seen the emergence of new *middleware* products designed to extract data from disparate legacy systems and put them in a compatible format. Examples include products and companies such as dbMotion, ICA CareAlign, Medicity MediTrust, Microsoft Amalga, Oracle HTB, and Orion Health. These technologies can play a role in making the transition from the current environment with little interoperability and document-based data exchange to an environment where data can be easily accessed and queried and assembled for a broad variety of uses.

The HITECH Act and Shifting Incentives

The discussion so far has highlighted barriers to the effective use of information technology in healthcare. Recent legislation, however, has started the Nation on what is potentially a new trajectory. In 2009, the *HITECH Act* (part of the American Recovery and Reinvestment Act, or ARRA) authorized expenditures on the order of $20 billion (with estimates in the range $9 billion to $27 billion) over five years to promote the adoption and use of EHR technologies that would be connected through a national health information network. The legislation sets forth a plan for the "meaningful use" of health IT to improve the quality of care and enable changes in delivery systems essential to healthcare reform.

The HITECH Act attempts to create incentives for all hospitals and eligible providers, not just those associated with large systems, to adopt and use electronic information. A centerpiece of the Act is to put in place strong financial incentives for hospitals and physicians to adopt and meaningfully use electronic health records. Physicians who adopt electronic records by 2014 can qualify for Medicare bonus payments of up to $44,000. Beginning in 2016, physicians who have not adopted electronic records will be penalized in the form of reduced Medicare reimbursements. Similarly, Medicaid providers can receive up to $63,750 over the five years. These payments and penalties depend on the provider meeting the requirements for meaningful use.

The definition of meaningful use under HITECH involves both ONC and CMS, but CMS is the principal rule-making body since payment will be linked to the reporting of meaningful use measures. The statute leaves CMS broad discretion, requiring only that the definition include e-prescribing, the ability to exchange information with other healthcare providers to improve care, and the reporting of clinical quality measures to CMS. With input from several Federal advisory committees, CMS has proposed to phase in meaningful use criteria in three stages. Stage 1 criteria, to take effect in 2011, focus on electronically capturing health information in a coded format, implementing decision support, sharing information with patients, testing the ability to exchange information, and initiating the reporting of clinical quality measures to CMS. Stage 2 criteria, to take effect in 2013, would require more robust exchange of information and other high value uses of EHRs. Stage 3 criteria, to take effect in 2015, would require physicians to demonstrate the use of EHR technology in ways that improve the outcomes of care. The broad goal is to gradually acclimate providers to workflow changes and practice improvement opportunities that, ideally, will accompany the adoption of technology.

Responsibility for implementing many other parts of the HITECH Act resides with the Office of the National Coordinator, discussed in the introductory chapter. In particular, ONC is responsible for developing policy guidance and a broader future vision for health IT. As we discuss below, it has already begun a series of important initiatives to further IT innovation and standards in a variety of areas. It also must work together with CMS and other Federal agencies. Indeed, as we now discuss, the division of authorities and responsibilities poses significant challenges.

Opportunities and Challenges for ONC and CMS

In the short time since the HITECH Act was signed, ONC has moved forward on several important initiatives. Perhaps the closest to this report is ONC's recasting of the Nationwide Health Information Network project. The NHIN is composed of standards and services that enable secure exchange of health information over the Internet, combined with a strong policy and trust framework that enables organizations to share health information with strong consent and governance to improve healthcare delivery while strongly protecting privacy and security. As we elaborate in Chapter Four, we believe that this initiative could benefit from a more aggressive focus on a universal, extensible exchange language and the development of associated national infrastructure.

The ONC has also moved forward in the important area of clinical decision support and enhancing usability of electronic record systems. With AHRQ and the Office of the Secretary, it has established a Federal "collaboratory" whose members now number more than 150 across more than 15 Federal agencies. The collaboratory has developed an inventory of federally supported CDS efforts, promoted sharing of best CDS practices, and identified needs and strategies that have resulted in new projects sponsored by ONC, AHRQ, and other agencies. Notable among these new projects is an effort to develop generalized representations of important medical logic (rules) that enables these rules to execute in the same way even if installed in different vendor systems. The ONC also has awarded a contract to the RAND Corporation to advance CDS. Work performed under the contract will advance the Nation toward a CDS knowledge repository, including the implementation of best practices and tools for sharing CDS interventions. It also will address the "alert fatigue" problem (the problem of too many inessential "pop-ups") by, for example, identifying those drug-drug interactions that are of highest priority. Another ONC initiative aimed at improving EHR usability is a collaboration with the National Institute of Standards and Technology (NIST) to develop usability testing programs that may become a part of EHR certification.

In addition to these efforts, ONC administers HITECH funding for Strategic Health IT Advanced Research Projects and has awarded four cooperative agreements totaling $60 million. An award to the University of Illinois at Urbana-Champaign addresses the challenges of developing security and risk mitigation policies and the technologies necessary to build and preserve the public trust as health IT systems become ubiquitous. An award to the University of Texas Health Science Center at Houston addresses the challenge of harnessing the power of health IT to integrate with, enhance, and support clinicians' reasoning and decision-making, rather than forcing them into a mode of thinking that is natural to machines but not to people. An award to Harvard University focuses on the development of a platform architecture that will facilitate substitutable applications—enabling the equivalent of the iTunes App Store for health—as well as supporting the electronic exchange and use of health information in a secure, private, and accurate manner. And an award to the Mayo Clinic College of Medicine focuses on strategies to make use of data that will be stored in EHRs for improving the overall quality of healthcare, while maintaining privacy and the security of the data.

CMS plays a rather different, yet pivotal, role in the national health IT effort, in large part due to its broader centrality in the Nation's healthcare system. As the Nation's largest payer, CMS has substantial leverage over healthcare providers. For example, it is often argued that the fee-for-service payment system used by CMS tends to reward volume over patient-centered goals like coordination and personalization. As noted above, some of the leading adopters of health IT, such as Kaiser and the VA, are systems with very different financial structures. Recent healthcare legislation (the Patient Protection and Affordable Care Act, or PPACA) supports many initiatives to reform healthcare payment and to advance CMS projects such as Medical Homes and Accountable Care Organizations, which aim to create incentives for coordination and more efficient care. As we discuss in Chapter Six these types of innovations can significantly complement health IT efforts.

Even more directly related to EHR adoption and use, CMS exercises substantial influence over the type of data that providers must collect. For instance, payment reforms based on quality of care measures require providers to collect and report these measures. This type of data plays a key role in current attempts to define meaningful use, where the idea is to create consensus "measures of quality," the collection of which can be translated into requirements for "meaningful use" incentive payments.

One concern with this approach, however, is that most quality measures depend on strict specifications that limit the flexibility to describe complex care coordination and functional outcome goals. Indeed, at this point, most are related only to individual specific conditions. The reason for this is that many of the validated, existing quality measures reflect medicine's traditional focus on treating particular illnesses, rather than on care coordination and health maintenance. Furthermore, most EHRs were designed around billing codes, not around rich clinical information that would give a more patient-centered view of the context and the true outcomes of care, especially as it occurs over longer periods of time. Legislation allows the Secretary of HHS to approve alternative pathways for these CMS payments. Thus, if more robust clinical data were available and easier for a sophisticated system to gather and report, the use of these data ought to be encouraged.

A second concern is the ability of CMS to receive and process any complex forms of clinical data. The historically underfunded IT infrastructure of CMS has not kept up with the constant new legislative demands for new programs, especially those requiring quality-of-care data for numerous value-based purchasing programs. The culture and structure of CMS, and the demanding time frames of each legislative mandate, have led to multiple separate data platforms and different administrative approaches to each of them. Thus, even within CMS, it is not currently possible to aggregate data, and (for example) physicians are required to double-enter specific codes to be eligible for quality incentive payments. Through certification standards for EHRs, ONC is trying to require that EHR vendors supply a short cut for physicians to do this, but even if this occurs, the specific data elements will not provide a full clinical picture of patient care, and will therefore provide limited constructive feedback to providers about areas for improvement and about the value of the aggregated data.

CMS has not been able to invest in the infrastructure needed for the enormous scope of its growing database and quality-of-care requirements. For example, a 2002-2003 data modernization plan that would integrate data across CMS programs was not funded until 2006, and now proceeds only slowly and incrementally. CMS recognizes that this work is far from complete. In planning stages, CMS has high level concepts for a transformed and modern payment system and an Enterprise Data Environment that could, if appropriately implemented, contribute to the goals of this report. However, lacking funding, implementation work has been stalled. Congress now recognizes that CMS must upgrade its own IT systems in order to handle clinical and other performance information and to ensure program integrity, and it has begun to authorize these important upgrades. Notably, PPACA charges CMS to accelerate work on the CMS Integrated Data Repository to incorporate into the model data from all Federal health programs. It also directs CMS to enter into data sharing agreements with the Department of Defense, the VHA, and the Social Security Administration.

While we have not investigated these issues further, it seems likely to us that a complete overhaul of CMS's IT infrastructure will be needed in the foreseeable future, not because of future health IT require- ments but simply for it to comply with existing legislative mandates. The National Research Council has recently begun work on a study of the CMS information system capability, with a preliminary report due by December 2010 and a final report due at the end of 2011. Because CMS's operational mission of payment processing must proceed without interruption, and because it is starting from a technologically outmoded base, it seems likely that any rebuilding of CMS's infrastructure will be a difficult and lengthy process.

This is an ideal time for the leadership of CMS to assess the overall capability of CMS to take advantage of modern computing and to set in place a plan to upgrade systems, break down silos, and reduce unnecessary barriers to state-of-the-art computing capability. Federal IT projects frequently incur cost overruns and schedule slippages,[38] and it will be a significant management challenge for CMS to avoid the fate of other government IT modernization and software development projects.[39, 40] There is clearly a danger that rapid and otherwise achievable progress in health IT, as envisioned by ONC and (even more aggressively) by this report, could be forestalled or derailed if it becomes tied to CMS's formidable IT challenges.[41] This must be avoided.

Conclusion

The state of health IT today can be summed up as a mix of "the good, the bad, and the ugly." This diversity, and especially the fact that perhaps 80 percent of physicians still do not use electronic records at all, except possibly for billing functions, creates a dilemma. Given the difficulty of bringing the healthcare system forward into the computer age, should we focus on small incremental steps? Or, having seen the remarkable adoption rates and advances of Internet-based technologies in other sectors, should we push for a more radical advance that risks leaving some providers behind?

Fortunately, there is a bridge between these two extremes. It is the fact that the Internet-based technologies create a platform for "disruptive innovation," meaning innovations that upset the status quo and can broadly expand markets. Cloud-based technologies and PHRs are potential examples of disruptive technologies in health IT. These types of technologies might allow the 80 percent of physicians who are non-digital to leapfrog some of the existing limitations of EHR systems directly into more modern technologies. Indeed this is precisely what we want to happen, and it is a direction in which ONC and CMS could concentrate their efforts.

In setting up a roadmap for how we might move in this direction, it is useful to specify a clear set of mid-term goals. These should include:

1. Universal access by clinicians and patients to the current frontier of EHR functionality.
2. A robust platform for developers to create user interfaces, decision support, storage, and archiving services that will be broadly available to end-users and will not require major capital investments.
3. Seamless, user-transparent, cross-organizational data exchange.
4. Innate, strong privacy protection on all data, both at rest and in transit.
5. Efficient means for the aggregation of de-identified data for public health and research purposes.

As already indicated in Chapter Two, we believe that there is *at least one* technical approach that can achieve all of these requirements. The approach that we favor, based on the exchange of metadatatagged data elements, is described in detail in the next chapter.

This chapter's bottom line: Despite success stories from some early adopters, the current level of IT use in healthcare is uninspiring.[42] Recent initiatives, particularly by ONC, are shifting the incentives and may stimulate substantial EHR adoption. But a substantial advance and concentrated focus are needed to develop a scalable, national health IT infrastructure. New technologies can assist in taking the required steps.

IV. Technology for an Integrated Health IT Ecosystem

Introduction

The current health IT landscape is dominated by enterprise systems based on proprietary formats. These systems lack ability to communicate and aggregate health information in the ways needed to serve patients, doctors, and researchers. The systems have been designed primarily to enable point-to-point communication of administrative information rather than clinical data. Importantly, the nature of current systems makes it difficult for innovators to develop new tools to improve the use of health information. There are few policies or governance models to drive innovations, such as research, advanced clinical decision support, or benchmarking. In short, there is no fuel for an ecosystem of economically self-sustaining healthcare innovation.

The overarching goal is to have a national health IT ecosystem in which every consumer, doctor, researcher, and institution has appropriate access to the information they need, and in which these groups are served by a vibrant market of innovators. At the end of the previous chapter, we listed a set of technical and market-related requirements for enabling this overarching goal. Here, we look at several possible technological approaches and describe in some detail an approach that, we think, has the greatest likelihood of rapid forward progress.

Earlier Models for Enabling Data Exchange

Over the last 20 years or so, an era dominated by vertically integrated, proprietary EHRs, one approach has been to seek to create *standardized health records*. Because the medical system has long relied on filling in paper records, it was natural to assume that exchange or reuse of data would be impossible without establishing standardized record formats that would be comparable across providers. However, we believe that any attempt to create a national health IT ecosystem based on standardized record formats is doomed to failure. First, there is too much diversity and incompatibility for any kind of *a priori* standard to emerge. With so many vested interests behind each historical system of recording health data, achieving a natural consolidation around one record format for any particular subset of data would be difficult, if not impossible. Second, systems based on fixed records are inherently limited in their functionality. Consider, for example, a health record in which all types of blood test information are always stored. When a new type of blood test is developed, it is difficult to expand the record to include it. Moreover, it is difficult to exchange only parts of such an electronic record according to a patient's choice (for example, blood glucose measures but not HIV status).

A second approach to health IT, spurred by the emergence of the Internet, has focused on service-oriented architecture (SOA) as a way to solve the problems inherent in standardized record formats. SOA essentially involves using software policies, practices, and frameworks to enable one user to access sets of "services" on another party's computers and data.[43] For example, two hospitals, using two different systems, might create bilateral arrangements that enable them to run "services" on each other's systems to execute transactions or access data. The approach could be expanded to small networks, and even to networks of networks.

As an analogy, one might consider two libraries with completely different systems for filing books. Each library's users have no idea how to find books in the other library. But if each library sets up a "service desk" with an actual librarian, then the other library's users can get what they need by lining up at the service desk for assistance. This analogy also makes clear one of the big limitations of SOAs, namely scalability. A library's own users can all be looking for books on the shelves at the same time; but users from the other library must queue for the librarian "service."

There have been extensive efforts to implement the above approaches in local and regional HIEs that seek to connect multiple organizations. By 2009, there were more than 190 HIE initiatives in the United States—although only about one-third were fully operational.[44] These HIEs report lower costs, improved outcomes, reduced staff time spent on process-oriented work, and increased data exchange—demonstrating the benefit of health information exchange. But despite these benefits, these approaches fall far short of what is needed. Most HIEs are based on standardized record formats or integrated care systems that cannot readily scale. Others link a range of proprietary systems. If a patient moves between two hospitals even within an HIE, critical tests done at the first hospital must often be repeated.

Most HIEs face the administrative burden of requiring adoption of legal agreements at each provider organization to share data. In addition, HIEs that began as pilot projects do not appear to be spreading or scaling up beyond their initial scope because they were launched without significant attention to long-term business models, a problem that the meaningful use incentives may not overcome. Most HIEs, moreover, are not currently interoperable across regions and markets to other HIEs, and thus remained closed and proprietary even as patients seek and require care outside their confines.[45] Because each HIE system is different, there is little incentive for entrepreneurs who make middleware and other innovative tools to serve this marketplace.

While such systems can surely be incrementally improved, we believe that such approaches will not solve the fundamental need for data to be universally accessed, integrated, and understood while also being protected. In a sector as fragmented and rapidly evolving as healthcare, we believe it is impossible to build a national implementation of SOA solutions and directories that could be used and scaled indefinitely into the future. (To draw a loose analogy, the approach is like trying to enable free trade among hundreds of entities by negotiating a huge number of bilateral trade agreements. Or it is like trying to promote dialog among speakers of a thousand different languages by training one million translators, each knowing a pair of tongues, instead of enabling them to speak a common language. The idea is laudable but impractical.) Moreover, the approaches will not overcome the barriers to entry for innovators wishing to develop new solutions. We believe that a steady supply of such innovators in the ecosystem is essential for increasing quality and decreasing cost.

Universal Exchange Using Metadata-Tagged Data Elements

The best way to achieve a national health IT ecosystem is to ensure that all electronic health systems can exchange data in a universal exchange language. The systems themselves could be designed in any manner desired — they could accommodate legacy systems that prevail or new recordkeeping systems and formats. The only requirement would be that the systems be able to send and receive data in the universal exchange language.

We believe that the natural *syntax* for such a universal exchange language will be some kind of extensible markup language (an *XML* variant, for example) capable of exchanging data from an unspecified number of (not necessarily harmonized) *semantic* realms. Such languages are structured as individual data elements, together with metadata that provide an annotation for each data element.

With some risk of oversimplifying, let us give an example. Imagine that an elderly patient has lived in several different cities and, over the years, has had mammograms done at various hospitals and clinics. Her physician now needs to retrieve images of her breast tissue over the previous decades to determine whether a current lump is of concern. In a health IT ecosystem where tagged data elements make up a universal language, the data elements the doctor could retrieve about this patient would include the mammograms themselves from all of the various places the patient has sought treatment regardless of provider network, geographic location, or whether the patient remembers them. The physician would be able to securely search for, retrieve, and display these privacy-protected data elements in much the way that web surfers retrieve results from a search engine when they type in a simple query.

What enables this result is the metadata attached to each of these data elements (mammograms), which would include (i) enough identifying information about the patient to allow the data to be located (not necessarily a universal patient identifier), (ii) privacy protection information—who may access the mammograms, either identified or de-identified, and for what purposes, (iii) the provenance of the data—the date, time, type of equipment used, personnel (physician, nurse, or technician), and so forth.

Most of the time, the metadata will not be needed by the physician; this information will be invisibly in the background. Occasionally, as in the case of a false positive or false negative in a particular image, the physician may want to dig deeper: The metadata will be there.

The metadata will also be important for researchers who may have access only to de identified data. They might use it, for example, to determine whether a certain type of imaging equipment for breast cancer is yielding excessive numbers of wrong diagnoses. This could result in improvements or recalls of particular devices and improvements in software.

Data Element Access Services

In the example above about retrieving multiple mammograms, we assumed more than simply a universal exchange language. We also assumed the existence of certain national infrastructure for *finding* health data, and for controlling access to it. (Importantly, though, we have *not* assumed a national repository for *storing* health data, which would be a more difficult and politically problematic issue.) We call this infrastructure, collectively, *data-element access services*. The services would include those associated with crawling, indexing, security, identity, *authentication, authorization,* and privacy. As proposed, these DEAS and their components would have no right to *use* the data being exchanged; in fact, they would probably not even see the data.[46]Rather, they would act much like today's web search engines, but with additional levels of responsibility for exposing only those data elements authorized by applicable privacy rules and policies (including a patient's persistent privacy choices) and only to authorized, authenticated users. A patient would have the right to restrict the types of data elements indexed at all, or could opt out of the DEAS completely (although such a choice might negatively impact that patient's future care). We discuss privacy protection and security in more detail in Chapter Five.

Today, when a user views a web page, the data that make up the various parts of the page (text, images, ads, audio, video, etc.) are dynamically aggregated in real time from numerous computers in a range of *physical* locations and are then presented to the user as a single *logical* entity: the web page being viewed. The individual elements are not routed through any central server or repository. Rather, a set of access services enables the browser to query many distant computers simultaneously. Similarly, for health IT, a query submitted to the data-element access services would result in the seamless, dynamic aggregation of all the data requested. For example, a doctor's request for patient information could involve an indexing system identifying all the physical locations on the network of the data; real-time aggregation of the data; and analysis, translation, and presentation by the software application that the doctor is using.

The health IT ecosystem we envision does not require the existence of a uniform patient identifier. Instead, it could use associations of intrinsic patient-related information to link the appropriate data to specific patients. This method is used now to create patient record locators within local closed systems and regional health exchanges, but as employed today, it can be plagued by human error.[47] Since an automated system can use many more than the two factors (such as name and birthdate) now often used, it can be correspondingly more accurate.[48] Indeed, "identity resolution" is an established technology, with commercial offerings available.[49] For greater accuracy and convenience in the record-keeping associations, some patients (e.g., those named "John Smith") might elect to index their records by an email address or a reference to a personal health record account, but this would be optional.

How should DEAS be brought into existence and operated? There are several viable options: Individual states (or self-formed groups of states) could establish and operate DEAS. Federal funds might be used in the manner of a "race to the top," to support the best state's proposals, or to create an additional interoperating and intercommunicating DEAS for use by Medicare providers. DEAS could be established in large health delivery networks (including those operated by the Federal Government, such as the Veterans Administration). They could emerge from a more aggressive push toward achieving interoperability among existing HIEs. Or, their growth could be left to the private sector, perhaps seeded by some start-up funds in response to requests for proposals.

As a matter of engineering, fewer DEAS providers is better, since communication between DEAS in response to queries is an additional overhead, but this must be weighed against socio-technical, governance, and policy forces favoring a more distributed network of DEAS.

In any case, all DEAS would need to be interoperable and intercommunicating in conformance to a single Federal standard, and would need to be audited for compliance with privacy and security policies. In response to a HITECH mandate, ONC has already begun a process for establishing governance of the NHIN.[50] This process might also explore how best to operate DEAS.

Advantages of the Tagged Data Element Approach

Because of its multiple advantages, we advocate a universal exchange mechanism for health IT that is based on tagged data elements in an extensible markup language. If there were another equally good solution, it should also be considered; we have collectively been unable to think of one.

Tagged data elements can be combined for a single patient to produce the equivalent of an EHR, and organized around the needs of that patient at the time of care. At the same time, the data can be analyzed and combined with links to other information to provide physicians with clinical decision support, delivering patient-specific information to their fingertips to make the best possible decision for a patient given all of the information available. Tagged data elements from aggregated populations can also be combined to analyze comparative effectiveness of aspects of healthcare and improve efficiency and quality.

Since the language of metadata-tagged data elements is extensible, not fixed, it can itself evolve in response to the development of new applications and new medical knowledge. As already mentioned, extensible exchange languages exist today and are already used within health IT in specialized niches— and are used widely in other sectors. A main finding of this report is that the time is ripe for such a language to be declared as a universal exchange language for health IT, and that doing so will catalyze a large number of immediate and longer term advances.

Tagged data elements can be extracted by special software (known as middleware) from existing clinical systems. Or they can be produced from enhanced versions of those systems, or by completely new and innovative applications. In this way, all data could be exchanged among all systems no matter the origin or internal record formats of the data, and without the necessity of replacing existing legacy software.

A universal data exchange language can scale up to any level. It can allow retrieval by patients and physicians of information from different providers, in different parts of the country, to improve safety and coordination. It can deal with the diversity and complexity of both the underlying business and clinical systems. New types of data and associated metadata can be added at any time, since new data elements do not have to fit into a particular format. Data can be converted to whatever form best supports their intended use, from clinical diagnosis to medical research. This approach can create a fully interoperable, less costly, more effective national health IT ecosystem.

The availability of a universal exchange language can dramatically accelerate the entry of third-party innovators, because they can create applications that rely on uniformly described data elements and can access a larger market. These new applications could include cloud-based subscription services for individual doctors, small healthcare practices, long-term care facilities, large practices, and hospitals to handle practice management (e.g., registration, scheduling, and billing); sophisticated medical systems (e.g., decision support, integrated lab ordering, medication management, allergy tracking); integrated medical-image management; *integration engines* to facilitate data exchanges with personal health records and other types of EHR in the cloud; and population health management (e.g., analytical tools for public health reporting, clinical research, and outcomes analysis).

The approach that we describe is consistent with existing market trends. Innovative companies are emerging that can access data from existing records and rearrange, store, and exchange the data as desired. Other companies are offering advanced software applications, information, and other services via the Internet. PHRs allow patients to store and monitor all of their health information and research their conditions using the full range of electronic resources.

The approach described does not require the creation of a uniform patient identifier or a national repository for healthcare data. The data, protected by strong *encryption,* can be stored on existing legacy systems or in the rapidly evolving "cloud" of distributed data stores.[51] Data involving a particular person can be stored in many different places and then aggregated, just as individual web pages are constructed from elements stored on many different computers. Specialized and secure search engines can crawl and index the metadata while actual access to the underlying data remains constrained by privacy protections.

This system can provide much greater security and privacy protection than can the current system. The attached metadata would describe the use and access provisions of the data, in accordance with law, policy, or the patient's privacy preferences where applicable. For example, in a circumstance where consumers give their consent for particular uses of their data and prohibit other uses, this information would be encoded in the metadata. For example, privacy restrictions embedded in the metadata could permit a physician to send a pharmacist the data required to fill a prescription and permit de-identified data to be used for clinical research, but restrict other uses of the data. Privacy considerations are discussed in greater detail in the following chapter.

This chapter's bottom line: A universal language for the exchange of health data is needed. An extensible markup language, where individual pieces of data can be tagged with context-setting metadata, is a straightforward solution and is superior to other proposed architectures.

V. Privacy and Security Considerations

Introduction

A key advantage of the tagged data element approach is that it will allow a more sophisticated privacy model, one where privacy rules, policies and applicable patient preferences are innately bound to each separate tagged data element and are enforced both by technology and by law. In this chapter, we briefly review the present situation as regards the privacy protection of medical information, and then explain the technology building blocks that will enable better approaches.

The Present Framework

American ambivalence about integrating health IT into the healthcare system is rooted in significant part to concerns about privacy and security. Even though a large majority of Americans believe that electronic health records will improve the coordination and quality of care,[52] many Americans also believe that there is a reasonable likelihood that unauthorized users will view such records.[53] For example, a 2006 survey for the Markle Foundation found that 88 percent of Americans believe digital records will reduce the number of unnecessary or repeated tests and procedures they undergo.[54] However, this survey also found that 80 percent of respondents were "very concerned" about theft or fraud, 77 percent were equally concerned about use of their records for marketing purposes, 56 percent were worried that employers would see their health records, and 53 percent expressed concerned that insurers would, too. A solution to this perceived privacy problem must underpin any overhaul of the medical-data ecosystem.

Concern about the privacy of medical data is predicated on a range of factors. First is the potential for discrimination—in access or economic terms—that might influence health insurance or employment. Second, for some consumers there is a sense that medical data are "different" than other personal data. From this perspective, financial data involve something an individual has, whereas medical data involve what an individual is. Third, the use of personal medical data by others is potentially exploitative. People may be comfortable with having their de-identified data used for beneficial purposes like disease research, but not if they believe that commercial interests may use such information to try to sell them something or otherwise exploit it. Finally, Americans harbor deep-seated fears about possible government access to *any* personal data.[55]

The HIPAA Privacy and Security Rules, which went into effect in 2003, establish a Federal floor of protections for health information. The Privacy Rule, as amended by HITECH, regulates the use and disclosure of identifiable health information held by health plans, including employer-sponsored; health clearinghouses; and health care providers who engage in certain administrative electronic transactions (such as submitting claims electronically (collectively called "covered entities") and their business associates.[56] In general terms, the Privacy Rule permits, but does not require, the disclosure of identifiable health information for treatment, payment and various health care operations without the express written permission of the patient. The Rule also permits the disclosure of identifiable health information for research and public health without patient permission, as long as a number of other specific, detailed conditions are met. As a Federal floor of protection, the Privacy Rule does not supersede state laws that are more stringent, such as those that require patient consent to exchange health information for treatment purposes.

The Need for Strong, Persistent Privacy Protections

To build and maintain the public's trust in health IT requires comprehensive privacy and security protections that are based on fair information practices and set clear rules on how patient data can be accessed, used and disclosed, and that are adequately enforced. An individual's right to have some meaningful choice in how their information is shared is one important component of a comprehensive set of protections. Where such choices are provided, either in law or by policy, they must be persistently honored.

A patient cannot make meaningful privacy choices unless he or she understands the flows and uses of information and can therefore make informed choices. That is not the reality today. In practice, the current consent model mandated by HIPAA rarely allows fully informed choices. HIPAA allows many common disclosures (for example, for treatment, payment, and healthcare operations) without any consent at all. Some other disclosures are allowed unless the patient specifically opts-out. Some particular transactional flows of data require patient approval, but patients have little real information about those flows or the uses to which they will be put. As seen by the patient, HIPAA protection is often little more than "sign here to acknowledge that you understand your rights under HIPAA," which, of course, few patients do.

Some provisions of HITECH are intended to remedy this situation and give patients more control over the flow of their health information. For example, patients now have the right to restrict a provider from disclosing identifiable health information to a health plan when the information relates to treatment for which the patient has paid out of pocket. In general, however, patients have limited control over the way their health information is shared.

An exchange language based on tagged data elements allows for privacy rules and policies to be more effectively implemented; it also allows for more finer grained individual privacy preferences to be more persistently honored[57], and it can potentially allow patients to make better informed, persistent privacy choices not just in the rush of a medical encounter but reflectively and in an informed manner. For example, in circumstances where patient consent is required by law, policy, or practice, as part of enrolling with a primary care physician, a new patient might be asked questions like these: Do you want your primary care physician to be able to see your complete medical record, including from other places that you have been treated in the past? Do you want this to be automatic for places where you may be treated in the future? Do you want your physician to be able to consult with other physicians and share relevant records with them at his or her discretion? If you are brought to a hospital emergency room, do you want them to be able to access your medical records without asking you? What if you are unconscious? Do you have a personal health record, and do you want your medical information to be automatically synchronized with it? Are there parts of your health history that you do not want disclosed to another doctor, such as treatment for mental illness? Do you want to be notified (or have your physician notified) when research using your data suggests new options for your own care?

There are pros and cons to the different possible answers to the questions in this example, and patients, in consultation with their physicians or other counselors, must understand these. For example, a physician must be able to know when a patient has chosen to withhold data and may not ethically be able to treat a patient who withholds medically necessary information. As a general principle, the more information that patients consent to make available in clinical situations, the more likely they are to benefit from better diagnosis and treatment options, especially those that may depend on their specific personal histories or genetic makeup.[58] Similarly, in sharing their information for research purposes, patients participate in a social contract that benefits everyone in general, but may also (with the help of an enabling health IT infrastructure) benefit themselves directly. Privacy and security protections need to be seen as enabling population research, not unnecessarily limiting it.

While face-to-face counseling on privacy choices should be available whenever choice is either required by law, policy or practice, most patients will probably educate themselves on the issues and make privacy choices through a web interface, where they will also be able to change their choices at any time. An important point is that, when patients have a meaningful opportunity to choose, a patient's choices will be persistent, that is, continuing until changed. Most patients ideally will have elected privacy choices at a time when they are healthy and competent. This is truer to the principal of informed consent than is a rushed signature at the time of a medical emergency, or when the patient's physical or mental competency is compromised.

Deleterious Effects on Medical Research and Care

The HIPAA Privacy and Security Rules, as well as sometimes more stringent state laws and regulations, were intended to enhance the privacy of health information. However, they have had the unintended consequence of freezing its exchangeablity. The complex mandates of both HIPAA and state laws and regulations leads organizations to equate protection to sequestration, with little or no provision for either access based on roles (for example, the needs of an emergency room physician) or for legitimate secondary uses of data (for example, epidemic tracking), although HIPAA itself actually does allow disclosures in many such cases.

Even before HITECH, some organizations' interpretations of HIPAA had proved detrimental to medical research and, potentially, care. For example, a 2005 study by the University of Michigan found that implementation of the HIPAA Privacy Rule was followed by a drop from 96 percent to 34 percent in the percentage of follow-up surveys completed by patients being monitored after a heart attack.[59] The report concluded that the Privacy Rule "significantly decreases the number of patients available for outcomes research and introduces selection bias in data collection for patient registries." Similarly, a 2006 study by the U.S. Government Accountability Office found that healthcare providers were "uncertain about their privacy responsibilities and often responded with an overly guarded approach to disclosing information to ensure compliance with the Privacy Rule.[60]

It seems likely that the modifications to HIPAA enacted in Subtitle D of the HITECH Act—in particular those that require covered entities to track all disclosures to associates[61]—will further stifle innovation in the health IT field while offering little additional real-world privacy protection. The limitations of HIPAA and the HITECH provisions (sometimes referred to as HIPAA II) should be reformulated so that they ensure both patient privacy and patient benefit from medical research, in a world where medical data are increasingly in electronic form and where there is a growing need for real-time or near-real-time aggregated data to improve healthcare. A recent report from the Institute of Medicine suggests that these policies need a major overhaul to enter the electronic age.[62]

Data Security: How Good Is Good Enough?

An exchange language based on tagged data elements enables a fine-grained model for addressing privacy, including honoring a patient's privacy preferences. However, this model is only as good as the level of security applied to the data itself. If an unauthorized user can compromise data security, and not get caught in doing so, then he can also compromise any patient privacy model.

In data security, the perfect is often very much the enemy of the good. It is important that criteria for electronic security measures not be overspecified to the point of impossibility. A useful point of comparison is the degree of security inherent in old-fashioned paper records stored in folders in a medical file room. These paper records are completely secure against large-scale, remote electronic "phishing" to sift through the records to find particular nuggets of information. File rooms seem *in practice* to be fairly secure against massive compromises even by physical means: breaking and entering to steal large numbers of paper medical files would not be a difficult criminal exploit, but it occurs virtually never.[63]

By contrast, paper records provide much less protection against unauthorized compromise (e.g., by copying) of the medical record of a single, targeted individual. We can infer from publicized cases that this happens regularly (for example, in the case of celebrities[64]). While private investigators cannot in most cases obtain a third party's medical records legally, they appear to have a significant ability to do so nonetheless. There is no reason to think that paper records are more secure than electronic records in the scenario of targeted individuals, since the exploit is typically enabled by suborning an insider with access to both paper and electronic records, or by social engineering (e.g., wearing a doctor's gown and walking into an unattended file room). In fact, paper records lack intrinsic security that is provided by even the most elementary electronic security protections. There is no way to tell if a paper record has been read or copied, for example. By contrast, an electronic system with basic authentication (by username and password) and auditing (of file accesses) preserves a record of who accessed what.

We can draw several conclusions: A health IT infrastructure needs to provide *significantly better* security than traditional paper records in all respects. It must be designed with *very strong* technical protection against remote, bulk attacks that compromise large numbers of records, because paper records do not have this vulnerability. The security of a single individual's information needs both technical protection and also protection by regulation and criminal law. Technical protection alone cannot prevent the suborning of otherwise authorized individuals, but it can greatly raise the bar by making them likely to get caught.

In today's healthcare sector, there is an astounding range of security practices in handling electronic data, ranging from excellent to poor. Importantly, there is little consistency in security practices. Sloppy practices have led to system failures at multiple levels, such as the massive compromise of personal data in a stolen laptop computer[65] or a burglarized hard disk drive.[66] In a well-designed system, as one example, it should be technically impossible for any individual to aggregate large numbers of records in an exportable format, and there should be multiple layers of real-time auditing to be sure that it is not in fact happening. We next turn to the question of whether it is possible to design appropriate protections for the privacy of electronic health records.

A Health IT Architecture for 21st Century Privacy and Security

We believe that a universal exchange language based on tagged data elements will allow the design of much better privacy and security protection than currently exists for either paper or electronic systems, for two principal reasons. First, the ability to tag an individual piece of data with privacy-related information, as part of its metadata, enhances privacy safeguards. Second, because tagged data element exchange protocols are designed to be efficient for the rapid exchange of small pieces of data, it is feasible to use security protocols that involve multiple exchanges of challenge and response. We illustrate these points in this and the next subsection.

How would this all work behind the scenes technically? Here we review briefly some of the technologies that can be combined to produce a well-designed system for protecting patient privacy, and indicate some of the design choices that will need to be made in creating such a system.

Encryption is the basic technology of making data completely unreadable unless it is brought into contact with a separate, smaller piece of data called the encryption *key*. Each piece of data can have its own key, or multiple pieces can have the same key. There can be several different keys that unlock the same data—for example, one for ordinary use and another (kept somewhere else) for rare emergencies.

A likely design decision would be that all patient information should always be encrypted either when *stored* or transmitted. Encrypting all "data at rest" (stored as on hard disk drives) protects against physical data breaches like misappropriation of hardware from healthcare IT data centers. Encrypting data "on the wire" (transmitted over networks), and authenticating the endpoints of every network connection, help defend against various network attacks, such as eavesdropping and misdirection of sensitive data to unauthorized parties.[67]

Another design decision could be to specify that a key for patient information is never stored (or even present) on the same computer system that holds its corresponding patient data. That would enforce technically that there be a *transaction* whenever data are to be used: the data must come from one computer system, and the key from another. The two computer systems can be physically distant, and managed by different organizations, so as to make insider threats much less likely. Transactions (which can themselves be encrypted) can be monitored and audited by a security infrastructure that is also independently managed.

Crucially, each encrypted datum carries metadata governing its specific use and access. These metadata are inseparable from the data and are inviolable, protected by a *digital signature.* While metadata are themselves likely encrypted (another design choice), their keys are, by design, known to an authorized set of secure search engines so that, for example, all the records of a particular patient can be located. However, the search engine has no access to the (differently encrypted) actual patient data.

Identity is also a crucial aspect of security. Determining the identity of a principal is commonly called authentication. Except for patient-consumers, all of the principals in the health IT system can be authenticated using physical credentials (such as smartcards), biometrics (such as fingerprints), and a secret such as a password. Requiring two of these three methods, a possible design choice, is termed "*two-factor authentication.*" Credentials could be issued to healthcare professionals by participating institutions and medical-certification agencies. Whenever data are accessed, an audit mechanism records the actions taken by principals, along with the information used to authorize those actions. Credentials can be revoked when necessary.

An authenticated principal has the right to perform actions in the system. Some rights might come from the identity of the principal (e.g., a patient has the right to see her records), while others might come from the role held by the principal (e.g., an emergency-room doctor has the right to see the medical record of an unconscious patient). Determining the rights of an authenticated principal is commonly called authorization. In the healthcare security system, a range of designated, authorized roles can be pre-consented, and anybody who presents the role credential will get appropriate access for a particular situation. This credential does not attach to the individual; it attaches to each specific role. For example, when an emergency-room doctor leaves for home, his or her role-based authorization is deactivated.

Finally, an audit mechanism records the actions taken by principals in the system along with the information used to authorize those actions. A secure audit mechanism must provide strong protection so that audit records cannot be tampered with or deleted. For example, an audit system must record any access, modification, or deletion of a patient's health records and any changes to the associated authorization policies. In case of an error in a patient's health record, the audit mechanism would reveal the principal who introduced the mistake and the authorization information for that access. Strong audit mechanisms can be implemented using cryptographic and other techniques.[68] Patients should have the right to review audit records pertaining to their data.

A well-designed combination of encryption, authentication, authorization, and, for research uses, de-identification can yield a health IT infrastructure that is secure, and where all principals are auditable. It can have strong protection against bulk data theft (for example, using real-time audit mechanisms on top of all the other controls), and be significantly better protected against insider threats to individual patient privacy than present paper or EHR-based systems. As already noted, technical security, no matter how effective, must also be augmented by administrative, civil, and criminal penalties. Because technical measures can never be perfect (especially against insider threats), it is ultimately these penalties that deter willful misuse by individuals or negligence by institutions. What well-designed technical measures can do is to make data compromises very difficult to perpetrate, and thus very rare.

Privacy Protection of Metadata-Tagged Data Elements

By way of example, let us look somewhat more closely at how the general technologies described above might be combined in an infrastructure based on tagged data elements. For the purposes of this example we will make an arbitrary set of design choices, not necessarily those that might be made after a careful systems study. Suppose that the data elements in question are, as in a previous example, the mammogram history of a particular patient, Abigail.

In a first scenario, suppose that Abigail's physician, Dr. Jones, queries to bring up all of Abigail's previous mammograms. The data element access services (DEAS) described in Chapter 4 first check that Dr. Jones has properly authenticated herself to the system and that she is in a role (e.g., primary care physician) that allows her to issue queries of this type. It then assembles (based on Abigail's name, date of birth, present and previous addresses, and so forth) a list of locations at which Abigail has medical records and has given prior consent for them to be locatable (assuming that rules or policies are in place requiring such consent).[69] If Abigail has consented to have the nature of her medical records also indexed (e.g., that some locations hold mammogram records, while others hold blood test records) then the list of locations can be pruned to a smaller number; otherwise the DEAS has no medical information and does no pruning. The DEAS now sends the locator information list (analogous to the web's "https://" universal record locators) to the EHR system on Dr. Jones's computer. That system, not the DEAS, then fetches the actual tagged data elements, each one containing a previous mammogram. It is important to note that the DEAS never has access to the mammograms themselves (the clinical data), and has access to even a description of the clinical data (the fact that it is a mammogram) only with patient consent. While most patients may elect a default choice that allows more efficient indexing and location of their records, the DEAS is designed to also serve (albeit with reduced efficiency) patients who choose to impose greater privacy restrictions on their data.

Can Abigail's mammogram images now be displayed? No, because they are still encrypted. For each data element, Dr. Jones's computer now queries another service of the DEAS for the required decryption keys. These requests include, again, Dr. Jones's own authentication data and role. They now also include the digitally signed (and therefore unforgeable) patient privacy preferences that accompany each mammogram as metadata. The DEAS examine whether Dr. Jones's credentials and role are consistent with Abigail's privacy choices. If they are, the DEAS send back the individual keys, and Dr. Jones's computer displays the mammograms. If they are not, then an explanatory message is sent and the mammograms are not displayed. In either case, the entire transaction is summarized in an audit record that goes, in real time, to a layer of security checking designed to look for anomalous signs of misuse. Such signs might include the collection of more patient records by a single supposed clinician than can plausibly make sense in that clinician's role, or a pattern of requests from a single facility for data on patients with whom they have no previous relationship and for whom they cannot supply any required evidence of patient interaction.

Notice that, in this and all scenarios, data and key are brought together only in the clinician's computer, and only for the purposes of immediate display; decrypted data are not replicated or permanently stored locally. Note also that the multiple data storage locations never had access to the keys, so compromise of their data, even by an insider with physical access, is impossible. Similarly, the DEAS that managed the keys never saw the data.

In a second scenario, suppose that an NIH researcher, Dr. Garcia, is studying the comparative effectiveness of two different mammography techniques. His credential and role identify him to the DEAS as authorized to receive only de-identified data from patients. When Dr. Garcia queries for data, he receives 100,000 locator records for mammograms meeting these criteria. However, these locator records are different from those returned to Dr. Jones's in the first scenario. Their unforgeable digital signature specifies that they may only be used to locate de-identified data. When Dr. Garcia's computer now sends out for the 100,000 mammograms (and their accompanying metadata), they come back de-identified, and they contain a digital signature that so certifies. Dr. Garcia's new DEAS queries for the individual decryption keys must now contain (i) his own authentication and role as researcher, (ii) the digitally signed privacy requirements and preferences (where applicable), and (iii) the certification that the data have already been de-identified. Only if everything matches do the DEAS provide Dr. Garcia's computer with the decryption key for each piece of de-identified data.

These examples are intended only as illustrations. In fact, the computer exchanges would be even more complicated than indicated. The fields of computer security and data protection are sophisticated and highly developed. While the web will continue to be full of reports of data compromises in badly designed systems, or systems subverted by bad management practices, there is no reason that a national health IT infrastructure should be designed and managed at less than state-of-the-art best practice. Our judgment is that such best practice can yield much better privacy and security for health IT than today's scattered approach, and also can be much more enabling of secondary data uses such as public health and research.

This chapter's bottom line: The tagged data element approach allows for a sophisticated, fine-grained model of implementing strong privacy controls (including honoring patient-controlled privacy preferences where applicable) and strong security protection.

VI. Economic and Regulatory Issues

Introduction

Many economic and regulatory steps need to be taken to realize the technological opportunities described in this report. This chapter offers a succinct discussion of some of the main issues. An important consideration here is that many aspects of health IT, particularly those associated with data exchange and aggregation, have "public good" characteristics. Because the benefits of a networked health infrastructure will be distributed widely, while costs are borne locally, market forces may fail to generate appropriate incentives for providers to invest in interoperability or to allow their data to be indexed and accessed. The public good nature of the problem calls for coordinated leadership to implement standards for interoperability and to enable indexing and retrieval of patient records. At the same time, policy makers need to create market conditions that reward information exchange, and enable market innovation to deliver the IT services and applications that can ultimately have a major effect on healthcare systems.

The technological approach described in Chapters Four and Five relies on two key elements. The first is the adoption by providers of interoperability standards that enable data to be shared across institutions. The second is the creation of network infrastructure and administration that enable distributed data to be indexed and accessed subject to appropriate data access restrictions. Both have the public good features mentioned above, in much the same way as investments in transportation or communications networks. We argue that Federal leadership exercised by ONC and CMS can play an important role in furthering both interoperability investments and network infrastructure development.

Standards and Incentives for Interoperability

As described in Chapter Four, one way to enable scalable data exchange and new application development is through the adoption of *standardized metadata* that enable patient data to be indexed, queried, transmitted, and re-assembled for different uses. This route to interoperability does not mean that every provider has to adopt a standard health record format or reconfigure its approach to inputting and managing patient records. Indeed, we pointed out that technology already exists and is offered by a variety of middleware providers that enables existing systems to become interoperable in this fashion.[70]

Nevertheless, the economic environment poses substantial roadblocks for investments in interoperability. There is not yet a recognized standard for health metadata, and healthcare organizations and technology providers considering adoption of a standard face a coordination problem. Even for the healthcare systems that are leaders in using information technology, there is little private incentive to focus on widespread interoperability unless other providers are making the same investment and there is a clear path toward productive data exchange.

Furthermore, the economic incentives of healthcare providers may not be strongly aligned with making patient data exchangeable. Healthcare providers with their current closed data systems may view their data at least partly as a proprietary strategic asset. A hospital may have an incentive to exchange data with local clinicians, improving patient care and tethering the clinicians more closely to the hospital. But the incentives become less clear if the hospital is contemplating exchanging data with competing hospitals or with providers who are not local and with whom it shares few patients.

The local and regional health information exchanges discussed in Chapter Three have gone some distance toward promoting data transfer between institutions. But these models in their current form do not use a tagged data element approach that enables parties to flexibly assemble and re-assemble data elements in different ways to respond to different types of patient encounters, address population questions, track drug effects or epidemics, or enable clinical research. Moreover, as described earlier, local and regional exchanges will not provide a clear route toward national interoperability if they adopt different standards or settle on different governance models for regulating data access.

Federal leadership, therefore, has a clear role to play in coordinating standards for health metadata and in creating economic incentives to adopt the standard. The definition of meaningful use and the rewards for being a meaningful user (and penalties for not being one) are powerful mechanisms for doing this. Current work on meaningful use already has begun to incorporate interoperability standards. The initial recommendations by the Health IT Standards Committee that were transmitted to ONC in March 2010 do describe data exchange standards that providers must adopt to qualify as meaningful users, but they are far less ambitious than the objectives laid out in this report. In the next chapter, we will make some specific recommendations for how these standards can be developed over time so that the lever of meaningful use can help promote an effective architecture for widespread data exchange.

We emphasize that there is a potential concern with pushing too many requirements into meaningful use. The concern is that this will create too onerous a burden for many healthcare providers, especially smaller physician offices that already may lag behind in adoption. However, the initial experience with meaningful use suggests that providers of the IT systems have a strong incentive to compete by ensuring that their products qualify under meaningful use. If meaningful use is expanded in a moderate way to require standardized metadata, technology providers likely will incorporate the standards into their products, and competition between technology firms will rapidly bring down the costs of middleware that will allow legacy systems to meet the standard.

Creating a Data Exchange Infrastructure

The second component to the technological model we have outlined is the network infrastructure that links healthcare providers, patients, labs, researchers, and other stakeholders and enables qualified users to query distributed data stored by partners in the network. In thinking about the development of such an infrastructure, an important economic point is that communication networks are very often characterized by increasing returns. One reason is user externalities: the more parties sharing data in a network, the more valuable is membership to any given party. A second is the spreading of fixed costs. On a per-member basis, the costs of creating an indexing and data retrieval service may be large if only a few providers are participating in the network, but many of the costs are fixed and hence decrease on a per-member basis with increasing participation.

Current efforts at health data networking are at relatively small scale. As we have described, they consist of local and regional health information exchanges and narrower initiatives between particular institutions (hospitals and affiliated local physicians, or Kaiser Permanente and the Veterans Health Administration). The ONC is offering important support to these efforts—for instance, through cooperative agreements with all 56 states and territories to lead and promote health information exchange and through its Beacon Community grants program, which provides funding to 17 communities to build systems by which hospitals, clinicians, and patients use technology to improve health.[71] An important strategic question, however, is whether local experimental projects are the appropriate approach if the end goal is a national infrastructure.

One way to achieve this is to ensure that pilot projects are scalable and employ sufficiently flexible and interoperable technology. There are several ways in which Federal agencies might take this approach. One possibility is that CMS, the VHA system, or the Department of Defense (DoD) could initiate scalable pilot exchanges using the type of tagged data element model described in Chapter Four. The ONC also could use its grant funding to promote exchanges with the same type of flexible and scalable architecture. Finally, meaningful use guidelines that require providers to expose certain data to qualified users over approved networks are a powerful incentive mechanism. We make specific recommendations about meaningful use in the final chapter.

Regardless of how the network takes shape, an essential piece of the approach described in Chapter Four is a service that would index data available to the network and allow approved parties to locate a patient's data and assemble data elements, in both cases subject to access regulations. We termed this the data element access services model. The provider or providers of these services do not need to physically possess or store patient records in a central repository. But the providing entity does need to index data stored in a distributed fashion and retrieve and transmit data elements in response to qualified user queries, in much the same way that Internet search engines index data on the web and assemble data elements in response to queries.

The economic and regulatory issues around this service require careful consideration. Because privacy concerns are paramount with patient data, any provider of indexing and retrieval services must be able to maintain the trust of patients and clinicians. While such services might evolve in response to market forces, it seems likely that, at a minimum, regulatory oversight by ONC will be important for preserving patient trust. For instance, one possible regulatory requirement might be that providers of indexing and retrieval services have no commercial interest in the data and operate in ways that seek to maximize benefits for patients and the general public.

Compared with the broader costs of health IT adoption, the costs of creating indexing and retrieval services are likely to be low provided that the network reaches sufficient scale. Nevertheless, if the entities providing the service are prohibited from making commercial use of the data, they will need a funding mechanism. One possibility would be for the Federal Government to provide initial funding. Ultimately a variety of models might work. Funding could come from small charges on queries or from a small fee assessed to insurers on the basis of their enrolled members. One potential advantage of having payers, rather than providers, be the source of funding is that payers are in the best position to pass the costs on to the general population, who ultimately will have to bear the costs for any technology investment. Also, obtaining funding from payers would not impose a direct financial burden on providers, labs, or pharmacies whose participation would be important for making the system valuable.

A Regulatory Structure for Data Access

The national health IT infrastructure we envision would also require a carefully considered system to control access and ensure patient consent. As described in Chapter Five, an important benefit of the tagged data element approach is that different data elements can have different levels of security. This means that a single system can allow a treating physician to access a complete patient record, a payer to access summary statistics from a physician, and a researcher to access de-identified data to enable clinical research on different treatments.

With a tiered system for data access, applications used by providers, patients, and researchers might be assigned roles that enable them to retrieve and use different types of data. Patients and providers could then consent to share data for certain purposes but perhaps not for others. For instance, they might consent to allow data to be accessed by other providers for direct clinical care or allow certain data elements to be accessed by researchers in other than de-identified form. But they might prohibit access to firms seeking to market pharmaceuticals unless they wanted to be targeted for advertising.

There are inherent trade-offs in formulating a regulatory policy for data access. Patients with privacy concerns and providers with an economic interest in maintaining proprietary data may prefer a tighter policy that limits data sharing and the ability of third parties to develop applications that make use of networked health data. On the other hand, such applications have the potential to yield substantial general benefits in terms of increasing the quality and consistency of care, informing patients, and facilitating research. In this sense, ensuring data access has some of the same public good aspects as interoperability and network investment—in particular, widespread general benefits and more targeted costs to privacy. It is important to keep this trade-off in mind in formulating regulatory policy.

Competition to Supply Technology

So far, we have focused mainly on the government's role in bringing about a national health data infrastructure. In our view, however, one of the advantages of moving in this direction is to invigorate market innovation. Indeed, developing a networked infrastructure likely will involve the expansion of several of the nascent technology markets mentioned in Chapter Three. These include the markets for cloud-based electronic record and clinical decision support systems tailored to smaller providers, for middleware products that allow disparate legacy systems to be made compatible, and for new applications that enable patients and providers to leverage newly available data.

The economic incentives created by ARRA have already generated substantial innovation and competition in cloud-based electronic record products. More than 300 companies are offering some form of EHR product for physicians. Competition among these companies already has led to more affordable systems and improved products. Some of the companies in this market also are offering guarantees that physicians who adopt their system will qualify for meaningful use payments.[72] These cloud-based products are likely to become increasingly powerful as data exchange increases because physicians in smaller practices will be able to take advantage of data integration and tools that currently are available only to physicians in large integrated practices. This market therefore has an important role in ensuring that all physicians and patients benefit from advances in health IT and data exchange.

As noted above, moving from the current system to a tagged data element architecture will require that existing systems be upgraded to achieve interoperability. If providers have sufficiently strong incentives to upgrade, either because of the benefits of data exchange or because of meaningful use requirements, large EHR vendors are likely to move to interoperability. For organizations with legacy systems, we observed earlier that middleware products already exist that can extract data from existing systems and put them into tagged element form. The products might also provide an alternative for clients of large vendors who want a competitively priced alternative to upgrading their current system. To ensure that providers have multiple options, it is important that Federal policies are consistent with this market remaining competitive and innovative.

One further technology issue that arises in envisioning the future path of health IT relates to the problem of data storage and aggregation. Providers using electronic records are currently adding roughly 80 megabytes of data per person per year.[73] This rate is likely to increase as imaging and genetic data expands over time. As datasets expand, there could be substantial efficiencies in archiving large amounts of data in aggregated repositories. Indeed, this may be one advantage of cloud-based products. As we emphasized earlier though, the networked environment we envision is not dependent on the *physical location* of data storage. In this sense, it is consistent with a scenario under which data remain physically located with individual providers and labs, and one where technology evolves to favor a regime where data are stored in more aggregated forms.

Innovation and Markets for Applications

Transforming large amounts of linked data into information that improves healthcare delivery and benefits patients and other stakeholders will require a sophisticated layer of application software. Chapter Three described in some detail the limitations of today's EHR systems that could be remedied with innovative applications. But because providers currently create and store data in many different ways and typically in closed systems, there is no common data "substrate" that application developers can use. Furthermore, short of individual time-consuming sales, there is no easy way to make data-centric products available to providers or patients.

An important advantage of the technological approach we have described is that it would enable new markets where firms compete to provide services and tools to patients, healthcare providers, payers, public health officials, and researchers. These tools might include products for patients to gather information about diseases using their personal health data, to input data from home health monitors, or to compare healthcare providers. Providers might benefit from improved tools for data entry, clinical decision support, or e-prescribing. Commercial products could also emerge to serve the general health system. For example, providers could benchmark their patient population and outcomes with peer provider organizations, enabling new forms of quality measurement.

Many of these tools might function by combining individual data with a broader reference database. Analogous products are common on the Internet. Map-based products that provide directions or help consumers locate businesses or services combine individual information (a person's location and interest) with an underlying population database (maps with GPS coordinates, traffic data, and inventories of businesses). Personal finance tools use a combination of individual financial data and broader publicly available data on financial markets. The Internet also offers a model for market creation. As increasing amounts of data have become available (real estate transaction prices, financial market data, search and browsing data, and social network data), companies have emerged to build applications that use the data and market these applications to consumers and businesses.

One set of applications might address the problems with usability of EHRs described in Chapter Three. One way to understand some of the usability challenges is that current systems do not necessarily format information in a way that reflects the decision-making and information-flow processes of medical care. The problem is acute if a patient is seen by several providers who have to exchange clinical notes or lab results in document form. A system based on tagged data elements, coupled with the ability to query remote data stored by other providers, can allow for new software products that would deliver the data that the physician and patient require at the point of care, including the ability to intelligently retrieve information for advanced clinical decision support (evidence-based guidelines, genetic information, clinical trial access, and so on).

Patients also stand to benefit from applications that would allow them to collect information on treatments and physicians or share information with those who have similar conditions. For example, with the infrastructure we have outlined, a patient with a new diagnosis might be able to search instantly for the local specialist who has seen the most patients with similar conditions and prognoses. While it is possible that many patients may be uninterested in this form of engagement or these types of tools and will prefer to rely on a physician's advice, there are likely to be a large set of patients, particularly those with chronic health problems, who are interested. Patients with chronic illnesses already benefit from being able to search the Web or share information through discussion boards and social networking sites. Many might have a strong interest in applications that would allow them to access information culled from underlying health records.

A further class of applications might help users compile and aggregate population-level data on health outcomes, physician performance, or population health. These applications could be geared toward provider organizations, insurance companies, public-health companies, and researchers, broadly defined.

The Broader Economics of Healthcare

A central point to keep in mind in thinking about the future of health IT is that the mere adoption of EHRs, and even the creation of a technological infrastructure for data exchange, is unlikely to have a truly transformative effect on the healthcare sector unless the appropriate economic incentives are in place to improve the quality of care and reduce costs. Indeed the same organizational and economic factors that have blunted the incentives to adopt IT will also affect the incentives of healthcare providers to use IT as they begin to adopt EHRs. In this sense, it is difficult to separate health IT issues from broader economic issues relating to the healthcare system. While addressing the broader economic structure of the healthcare system is far beyond the scope of this report, it is useful to highlight a few of the issues and mention some current Federal initiatives that may complement health IT efforts.

To see the issues we have in mind, consider the common claim that EHRs can eliminate duplication and reduce healthcare costs. While it may be true that, for instance, networked EHRs could allow access to recent lab tests, one also needs to remember that in the healthcare system, one person's costs are another person's income. There often can be a fine line between duplication and a useful safeguard, and to the extent that providers have strong financial incentives pushing in one direction, the mere installation of IT systems may not reverse behavior.

Taking this example up a level, it is widely understood that the dominant fee-for-service model does not provide much incentive to streamline care, and also that the fragmented organizational structure of healthcare makes it challenging to move away from this model, because each small practice or hospital is a "tub on its own bottom" financially and therefore is not rewarded for interactions with other providers. This puts some of the major potential benefits of health IT, such as the ability to coordinate care across physicians, or to share and aggregate data from clinical encounters, somewhat at odds with the prevailing economics of the healthcare system. From this perspective, it is clear that the vision of health IT we have described needs to be supplemented by a broader set of reforms in payment and healthcare organization to realize the full potential of these technologies.

Several of the CMS initiatives funded under the Patient Protection and Affordable Care Act (PPACA) are notable in this regard, because they potentially complement health IT efforts. One such initiative is the primary care medical home model, which would put the patient and primary care physician at the center of a virtual organization that is paid a fee to coordinate all care the patient receives from specialists and other providers. In this model, the primary care physician would need to be able to exchange patient information seamlessly with other providers and assemble a complete record of the patient to successfully coordinate care. Another is the accountable care organization model, which would group hospitals and physicians into larger organizations that would contract with payers to care for an entire population. In this model, physicians and hospitals would need to share patient data and information to coordinate care, reduce unnecessary emergency room and hospital use, engage patients and families to enhance self-care, and track patient outcomes in a continuous manner. Both of these models would seem to require the type of coordination and data exchange that health IT can provide.

Advances in health IT are also likely to facilitate many proposed innovations in healthcare payment. Many of these innovations, and particularly those authorized as pilots under the PPACA, revolve around either pay-for-performance or bundled payments. With pay-for-performance, providers would be rewarded or penalized for patient outcomes relative to some quality benchmark. Bundled, or episode-based, payments would shift payment away from fee for service toward payment for all treatment following a diagnosis or for a set of procedures and subsequent care.

Estimating Costs

PCAST has not performed a detailed analysis of the system-wide costs associated with implementing the recommendations of this report. However, some general comments on costs are in order here. Overall, the approach recommended in this report is expected to *improve* healthcare quality, *decrease* the cost of health IT systems (due to increased competition) and lay the foundation for systemic reforms to increase the efficiency of healthcare. These benefits are likely to be distributed widely throughout the healthcare system and persist over a long period of time. The transition costs to achieve these savings are expected to be small, both compared to the broad societal benefits and to the overall $20 billion scale of the Federal health IT effort. These costs will be borne more narrowly, at least initially, by EHR vendors, healthcare providers, and government agencies. It is useful to distinguish several components of cost:

1) An initial cost for developing standards for the universal exchange language and its associated privacy and security protocols. Based on this group's examination of a range of analogous activities from other sectors of the economy and a survey of the literature and colleagues, we estimate the engineering cost of developing the actual standards to be in the range of $20 million to $40 million.
2) For healthcare providers with installed EHR systems, a cost to upgrade their systems, or to add middleware, so as to enable the exchange of data by means of the new protocols. Based on the current cost of middleware products, we estimate the incremental cost might be 5 to10 percent of providers' current EHR costs. On the other hand, this estimate may be overstated, because a nationwide move to adopt the new communication protocol would likely result in significant competition to supply upgrade products, which would place price discipline on incumbent EHR providers. We estimate that to upgrade their products, existing EHR vendors might have to make one-time engineering investments on the order of $5 million to $20 million per vendor, based on estimates of private investment in companies now offering products with similar levels of controls and privacy. The duplication inherent in these costs can be reduced by the Federal Government developing, and putting into the public domain, reference implementations for key processes (such as security functions).
3) For healthcare providers with no current EHR system, the additional cost associated with the new requirements of the universal exchange language. We expect this cost

to be minimal or absent. The proposed approach will likely to result in a more competitive and innovative market for EHR solutions, for example cloud-based products that are well-suited for smaller providers.

4) Capital and operating costs to the government associated with the infrastructure for indexing and searching patient healthcare data, and for related trusted security processes. Here, we note that multiple companies such as Google, Microsoft, Yahoo, Baidu, and some that preceded them, have made private investments in building and provisioning search systems for the entire Internet, which dwarfs the quantity of information in health IT. We estimate the proposed costs as being on the order of \$100 million to \$300 million per year, probably ramping up from the lower figure as the use of these services ramps up correspondingly, producing greater national cost savings. Included in the costs is an assumption of 0.1 GB per person, which would today be \$0.20 per person per year, a total of \$62 million in storage costs. One possibility is that the Federal government would bear the cost for the initial capital investment, and that the costs ultimately would be borne by either all users of the service, or by healthcare payers, including the government in its role as a payer.

This chapter's bottom line: Some aspects of the new health IT infrastructure will enable new, competitive, entrepreneurial markets. Some other aspects are "public goods" and will require government leadership. The benefits of health IT affect, and are affected by, other aspects of healthcare reform, especially payment models.

VII. Health Data and the Research Opportunity

Introduction

Today, most information about the effectiveness of therapies such as drugs derives from small-scale observations of a handful of patients (often a few hundred, sometimes fewer) in clinical studies. The most convincing clinical studies incorporate design elements, such as randomization of subjects to alternative treatments, to reduce the impact of unmeasured confounders on the treatment effect. These studies are appropriately considered to produce the highest quality evidence regarding a particular agent's efficacy, but they also suffer from well-recognized problems.

Efficacy, not effectiveness: Clinical research studies usually focus on highly selected and often nonrepresentative patients. They are designed to detect differences in the main outcome of interest, which means they are often too small to pick up less common but potentially important outcomes (such as serious adverse events) and are too brief to capture fully the long-term consequences of different treatment strategies.

For efficiency's sake, the studies often exclude patients with complex medical histories or many illnesses. This is problematic in that the treatments are needed by patients with complex illnesses where multiple different conditions make the range of choices greater than the usually simple comparison of a single trial.

Out of date before they are even finished: Today's clinical research studies are not carried out in real time. Instead, they take years to design, fund, launch, and complete. Sometimes, by the time they are completed the question under investigation is obsolete. For instance, it is quite common for multiple clinical trials in cancer to be occurring simultaneously. New drugs can then be approved that have never been compared with each other, so the physician and patient do not have any way of knowing which is best. They only know that each is better than some other drug that is no longer used.

Burdensome and costly: Today's clinical research enterprise is, at best, a sidecar loosely tethered to the clinical care enterprise. What is done in clinical research has its own expense structure and funding stream. The oversight of research is separate and apart from the oversight for clinical care. Its participants—both patients and investigators—are involved in sometimes redundant or repetitive activities. For instance, data often are collected twice for patients in clinical research studies: once for the patient's chart, and again for the research database.

Narrow focus: Most research focuses on a narrow set of questions regarding therapeutic choices. Yet many important questions in healthcare stretch far beyond the choice between drug A or drug B. For example, healthcare research needs to evaluate operational aspects of the delivery system and evaluate arrays of therapeutic choices side by side. Ideas for new directions for research can and should come from observations about health trends independent of specific hypotheses.

The Potential for Real-Time, Real-World, and Comprehensive Data

Numerous questions that clinical research is poor at addressing today could be answered using large datasets gathered through ongoing medical care, particularly if the data were available in near real time. A list of questions that could be addressed illustrates the promise.

Syndromic surveillance and public health monitoring: Our infrastructure for monitoring public health is spotty and slow, depending on individual offices reporting data locally or regionally. Health IT and real-time data on the use of the healthcare system have the potential to address this deficiency. Today, the ability to follow cancer trends, asthma and other environmentally sensitive conditions, antibiotic resistance, or flu-like symptoms requires additional infrastructures layered on top of the healthcare delivery system (such as cancer registries or emergency room reporting).These infrastructures are costly and incomplete. In many cases, they also are unable to produce details related to the entire population (the denominator) against which this information should be compared.

Routine collection of data could eliminate redundancy, be far more comprehensive, and overcome the denominator problem. Case ascertainment (such as detecting new cases of cancer or new cases of antibiotic resistance) would grow naturally out of data capture during routine clinical care. Moreover, the denominator (or denominators) would grow out of the same resource. For instance, it would be straightforward to assess the prevalence of antibiotic resistance across all cultures of a certain bacterium in a geographic area during a certain period of time. Those data could be married to data on prescriptions of different antibiotics in ways that cannot be achieved today.

There are working examples of such real-time data collection. New York City monitors pharmacy purchases as a way of capturing early signs of flu-like symptoms.[74] This activity is important for routine decisions about vaccinations and also for such factors as bio-terrorism preparedness. Current search engines also can identify a flurry of inquiries about flu, but they cannot identify whether the queries resulted from symptoms or from media exposure.

Adverse event monitoring: An ongoing concern for drug and device safety is the lack of a routine system of data collection for adverse events. The Food and Drug Administration mostly relies on *ad hoc* reporting of events. It does not have a good way to estimate the relative frequency of atypical events among all patients exposed to a drug or device or to separate association from causation. With extensive use of health IT and aggregated data, the data would be sufficiently rich to identify patterns and to separate events caused by particular drugs and devices from those that occur purely by coincidence.

Many examples of such event detection exist. The most frequently cited is the linking of Vioxx to cardiovascular events—something achieved through analyses of data captured by Kaiser Permanente and reported by several insurers as well.[75] Other examples include the detection of cardiovascular complications associated with the diabetes drug Avandia and with several calcium channel blockers used for treating high blood pressure.[76] Yet these represent relatively rare cases of adverse events detected through clinical databases. Other serious adverse events, such as those observed in randomized trials measuring the effect of erythropoeisis stimulating agents on cancer progression, were not detected in administrative data even though the effects were large, because there was not enough clinical detail in the information. This limitation could be overcome by greater data availability.

Assessments of dissemination and utilization: The gap between knowledge and the delivery of care, branded as the "quality chasm" by the Institute of Medicine a decade ago, remains a serious concern. The shortfalls disproportionately affect members of minority groups and individuals who lack insurance.[77] Currently, numerous redundant and sometimes conflicting systems aim to monitor utilization and quality as a way to mitigate these problems. Through programs such as quality measurement and reporting, chart review, and auditing, providers are increasingly being asked to report on what they are doing. This set of approaches, although conceptually attractive, has many problems. Any quality measurement collection involves large costs and burden. It also involves choosing the quality measures before creating a structure to capture the measures, which means both that the domains of quality that can be assessed are logistically limited and that the speed of change is sub-optimal.

The potential of data to monitor quality and the use of evidence-based approaches is immense. At scale, health IT will provide insight into the quality of care in all settings without actually having to design systems to report a particular element. The initial standards for meaningful use emphasize this potential benefit. If clinical systems capture sufficient data about patients, including both their eligibility for particular treatments and their contraindications, along with physician orders, e-prescriptions, and other delivery data, continuous quality monitoring and feedback could become part of routine care rather than the add-on it is today.

Comparative effectiveness research: Perhaps the greatest potential of the data that can be captured using health IT lies in the potential to fuel comparative studies of diagnostic and therapeutic approaches. Comparing treatment and management approaches in a way that can easily be accessed by both physicians and patients could improve patient outcomes and reduce healthcare spending. Funding for comparative effectiveness research is already growing. Electronic health information, in the easily accessible form enabled by metadata-tagged data element collection, aggregation, and security standards, would enable this kind of research to advance much more rapidly than with the traditional, institutional EHR model.

Supporting Research Uses

The uses described above, although they all hinge on data collected through EHRs, require somewhat different types of data, falling broadly into one of three categories: Effective *syndromic surveillance* and other public health monitoring could be achieved through collection of data that are already regularly recorded in patient charts but are not currently aggregated. *Separation of adverse events from coincidence and ascertainment of quality measures* may require more detailed information than is currently routinely captured in most patient charts today, but likely possible to capture within the system that we envisage. However, *comparative effectiveness studies*, particularly those that build in some experimental design or require additional data elements or assessments, would require more data than are routinely captured and also would require a framework of two-way interaction with the clinician and patient. We will illustrate this in an example below. And there are many other types of clinical research, not just clinical trials, in which two-way interactions between research and clinicians are desirable.

Methodological issues will need to be considered as data from EHRs become available for research studies of increasing sophistication. Practicing physicians are busy, not necessarily trained in research, and not always ideal collectors of patient data for research. Patients, exercising their right to opt in or out of studies, will cause data to be collected from incomplete, or incompletely defined, populations. Effects like these complicate the design and validation of research results. But the availability of data in quantities orders of magnitude larger than today will allow subtle and sophisticated experimental designs, more than compensating, we think, for the data's complexities.

Linking Patients to Clinical Studies

To see the potential for interactive data collection in EHRs to lead to the enrollment of patients in clinical trials, consider an oncologist who, upon seeing a patient with a new diagnosis of cancer, could be asked by the interactive program to upload detailed information about disease type, stage, other conditions, and performance status. Depending on that information, lists of eligible ongoing studies could be presented to the treating physician and patient, and enrollment in the study could occur during that visit. As an intermediate step, a more intensive data collection could be initiated, along with patient enrollment into a registry when enriched data are needed to address a particular question.

The value of such a system is clear. More information generated in clinical care could be used to accelerate learning, and many biases that exist in observational data could be overcome through the use of several types of experimental designs (such as randomization or block assignment). Providers and the patients would know all of the available opportunities to participate in clinical trials, and the physician could manage the patient through the process, with real-time data exchange to and from the research team. Not all providers would be authorized investigators in any trial, but electronic access to every available study would include the real-time ability to query the study about its appropriateness for the interested patient and any additional information. Much of this could be done without the patient having to transfer care to another provider.

Real-Time Patient Benefits from Comparative Effectiveness Research

Making patient clinical data available to researchers clearly has long-range benefits to patients. Until now, this has been a linear process with a timescale of years, since it requires performing the research, submitting it for peer review, publication, and ultimately the adoption of new clinical practices that benefit future patients.

Health IT can make it possible to get benefits to patients much faster. Indeed, patients could benefit directly from a research study to which they are concurrently contributing.

If patient progress and outcomes were routinely captured in data and made available in near real time, partial data can be used in sophisticated ways to assign treatments to new patients in optimal ways. These data also could be used to personalize treatment for patients already enrolled in a study.

A patient-physician interaction in an *adaptive comparative study* might proceed along these lines:

1) Using the physician's diagnosis, the physician's computer identifies a comparative effectiveness study relevant to the patient's condition and advises the physician.
2) The physician asks the patient whether he is interested in participating. The patient is advised that, by participating, he will receive a treatment recommendation based on, literally, today's best weighted judgment of all the accumulated data. However, the recommended treatment might not be the brand name drug that he expects.
3) agrees to participate in the study.
4) Through the physician's computer and the physician, the patient is asked if he wants to allow the study to access his personal genotype data, in which case a more personalized treatment recommendation might be made.
5) The patient agrees to this.
6) The study recommends a treatment, for example a prescription which is sent through the physician's computer (with patient and physician concurrence) to the patient's local pharmacy.

This example demonstrates a synergistic combination of three health IT opportunities, each potentially revolutionary. The first is real-time decision support to the physician based on evidence-driven best practice. The second is the real-time interaction of that decision support with completely current clinical data, without months or years of lag. The third is seamless integration of the clinical setting with the enrollment of patients into the clinical and comparative studies that will generate the next round of new data. Importantly, because these studies are adaptive (that is, they assign patients to treatments not arbitrarily, but rather based on the partial accumulated study data), they are consistent with the physician's duty to give each patient the treatment believed to be best for him or her on the basis of the most current evidence.[81]

Committing to only one level of data collection at a national level would be a mistake. A lot can be achieved based on clinical data gathered during routine care only, while some research requires additional data gathered during healthcare encounters. Other research may require experimental designs that entail additional steps such as informed consent, data categorization, follow-up questionnaires, and the like. To accommodate different levels of data collection, the infrastructure should be designed while considering the tradeoffs of collecting research-quality data against possible burdens. These burdens include a higher level of training for the providers involved and possible additional costs and processes required for high-quality research data, but the burdens can be limited and the advantages enhanced with access to a tagged data element environment. The implied trade-offs are matters of policy, to be codified only after careful consultation with all stakeholders, and to be justified not by the abstract desirability of research, but by explicit consideration of how research feeds back to better patient care.

Some opportunities and challenges in observational data: Observational data first uncovered the cardiovascular side effects of Vioxx, long before randomized trials demonstrated the same findings. Likewise, the apparent benefits of some unusually effective cancer treatments, such as Gleevec for chronic myelogenous leukemia, were apparent based on outcomes of studies using single specified therapies, well before randomized trials documented the actual size of the beneficial effect.[78] Yet observational studies can be hindered by biases that can be hard to detect, and sometimes findings are disproved by randomized trials or observational studies that contain more granular data. For instance, numerous observational cohort studies suggested that beta-carotene supplementation would reduce the risk of developing lung cancer, but randomized trials of the intervention showed the opposite effect.[79] A recent observational analysis of radiation treatment for women with DCIS (ductal carcinoma in situ, an early stage breast cancer) suggested that delays in radiation reduced overall survival, even though the underlying disease has a very low mortality rate and randomized trials of radiation for it had shown no mortality benefit.[80] The potential, and the limitations, are one motivator for providing an infrastructure that will eventually allow more than one approach to EHR-driven research.

This chapter's bottom line: A national health IT infrastructure will enable new kinds of research and will also create opportunities for the faster coupling of research to clinical practice.

VIII. GUIDANCE TO AGENCIES

Introduction

In this final chapter, we discuss what needs to be done if rapid progress toward the realization of a national health IT infrastructure is to be achieved. Because of the complexity of the issues, we give recommendations at several levels of specificity. First, as an example, we sketch a possible roadmap for getting all the way to the transformative future that we envision. Next, in narrative format, we give some overall short-term guidance relevant to the two key agencies, ONC and CMS. In the next chapter, we give a list of specific recommendations to several agencies that can (and, we think, should) be tracked by senior policy makers within the Executive Office of the President as to progress achieved.

A Feasible Roadmap to the Future

An important feature of the tagged data element model advocated in this report is that there is a natural transition path from present EHRs and from existing demonstrations of information exchange. As an illustration, we sketch a possible way—though by no means the only possible way—in which that transition might unfold. Key to this roadmap is its leveraging of universal data exchange, and the network effect, to spur EHR adoption.

First, HHS would define by regulation the most basic features of the tagged data element exchange. This would include the specification of an extensible markup language, most likely a variant of the existing language XML. ONC's clinical document architecture standard is important foundational work for this. However, additional focus is needed on aspects that relate to data transmission, to innate privacy features, and (perhaps most importantly) to facilitating the disaggregation of complex records into the smallest possible data elements, suitable for use by a broad range of new health IT products in a new, entrepreneurial marketplace. The universal exchange language is more than just an extensible wrapper for the exchange of documents, each in its own fixed format. It needs to facilitate (if not directly require) the exposure of the underlying semantics of individual data elements for new uses, including many not anticipated by the original data producer.

Also defined from the start would be a minimal initial set of requirements for the metadata that will accompany each piece of data. These might include, for example, the patient's name and birthdate, the applicable privacy rules and policies, including any patient's pre-consented privacy choices (e.g., "data may be used in research but only when fully de-identified"), an identifier of the originating physician or institution, a provenance within that institution (for example, a reference to a type of equipment or standard clinical procedure), and a time-stamp. Since the language is extensible, only a minimal set of metadata needs to be standardized at this stage; more will naturally evolve at later stages of adoption or as features added by individual software vendors.

A part of the specified metadata—for example, the patient name and birthdate—would be specified as "indexable" items that are made visible to authorized data element access services for indexing and data locating as they become available in stages of the transition.

Next, ONC and existing standards groups would publish mappings of existing vocabularies and content standards (for example, the HL-7 vocabulary standards for electronic exchange of healthcare information[82] and the ICD-9 and ICD-10 international disease classifications[83]) into the adopted markup language.[84] This straightforward step immediately expands the semantically meaningful realm of tagged data exchanges to include data that are coded in these existing standards. It incorporates these standards into the new architecture, leveraging the work done by thousands of people for decades.

In parallel, vendors of existing EHRs would be encouraged to rapidly publish mappings of their existing exchange mechanisms into the extensible markup language. For example, if a product is now able to exchange prescriptions, whole medical records, or other information, the vendor should easily be able to map that exchange at the existing level of aggregation into the markup language. This is only a first step toward an infrastructure of fully tagged data elements, because the individual data units are not yet the smallest pieces that make sense to exchange and aggregate. However, it is an important step, because it immediately allows the development of middleware that is able to exchange and display information from multiple vendor systems. It also is an important first step toward creating the kind of competitive marketplace that we envision. Data from patient-controlled personal health records can likewise easily be mapped into the new framework.

Many, if not all, of the meaningful use exchanges that are posited for the near future can and should also be mapped into exchanges of tagged elements within the framework of the markup language. Also important is a standard metadata markup for physicians' clinical summary records and case progress notes. There is no requirement at this stage for any exotic natural language processing or coding of these items. Their textual contents are exchangeable data elements in their own right whose exchange can add valuable clinical context.

After only these steps, we would already begin to see the value added of a single framework for tagged data element exchanges. At this point in the transition, the data are not yet in the smallest pieces that make sense and are not yet accompanied by all the metadata that will ultimately be needed. But the data will already have become universally exchangeable and universally privacy-protected, and the data will already incorporate large, widely recognized semantic realms. This is where the power of emergent markets, and the network effect, will first be felt.

Next in the transition sequence, ONC would define standards for the surfacing of metadata for use by the data element access services—that is, for finding and requesting patient clinical data (e.g., data relevant to a particular patient who presents in an emergency room) and also research data (e.g., anonymized data for a particular study by a state public health agency). In parallel, ONC (or another agency under ONC's policy direction) would would encourage the development of intercommunicating and interoperable DEAS. The DEAS will initially be much like any of today's web search engines, but they will be secure and specialized to privacy-protected data exchanges within the health network.

This is the point at which patients and clinicians would see tangible benefits from "putting the patient back together." Aided by new software applications, physicians will start to see tailored, unified views of all of a patient's interactions with the healthcare system, seamless across institutional and geographical boundaries.

In parallel, both as the market for health IT becomes more competitive and also to meet new government or payer requirements, vendors of existing EHRs would start to break down their data exchanges into smaller, more elemental units. For example, a regulatory requirement for metadata that includes the model and calibration of the instrument used in a specific lab test will cause the data to be exposed as tagged elements, rather than as part of an unwieldy integrated EHR. If there are new entrants into the EHR business, they should see a competitive advantage in producing systems that use metadata-tagged data elements by original design. At the same time, existing vendors, or unrelated middleware vendors, will provide add-on software to expose existing EMR information in an exchange interface where it appears as tagged data elements, regardless of how it is internally represented. The feasibility of such middleware is demonstrated by the fact that, as we have noted, in special cases it already exists today.

Over time, deliberatively and by appropriate processes, ONC and CMS would require (by means of the meaningful use or certification regulatory mechanisms) that smaller meaningful units of tagged data, and more extensive metadata tagging, be exposed at the interface, so as to be encouraging the development of new software applications and new benefits to the physician and patient. We will have gotten to this point by incorporating into the new framework, and then incrementally upgrading, health IT systems that exist today. Also, by creating a universal framework, new markets will be created for innovative software applications whose internal representations of the data, and thus capabilities, may be amazingly different from those available today.

Guidance on Necessary Design Choices

The development of a complex information infrastructure, such as that required for health IT, requires many design choices at many levels, and with appropriate ordering in time. Early conceptual design choices may have large, and even unanticipated, effects on later implementation-related choices. An important concept is that every choice *limits* the possible design space of subsequent choices. Sometimes this is desirable, because it forces convergence to desired goals. Other times, and especially early in the design process, it is important that design choices *preserve* a wide range of subsequent design options. Good systems design consists of finding the golden path between the extremes.

One often hears it said that "government should not dictate IT architectures," and we agree. The word "architecture" implies a series of decisions extending far down into the design process. What government *does* need to dictate, or at least facilitate the early standardization of, are those early design choices that will enable interoperability. These choices do not specify architectures, but rather "high-level protocols," or "data exchange languages," or even just common ways of thinking about the problem from a global perspective. Here government, both by its convening powers and by its regulatory authorities, has a crucial role to play, for the reasons already discussed in Chapter Six.[85]

ONC leadership recognizes (as do we) that complete interoperability in the entirety of the domain of healthcare is a massive undertaking. This has led to an approach that is iterative and incremental, focused on producing the specific, limited solutions that bring the greatest immediate value. The problem with this seemingly sensible approach is that it can result in a set of ad hoc solutions, rather than in high-level design decisions that could be both convergent and preserving of a wide range of possible subsequent design options. A key example, previously discussed, is the rapid establishment of a universal, extensible exchange language. As a more general statement, we think that ONC needs to augment its current multifaceted approach with a process that can generate design choices at a national level that are carefully balanced between the goals of convergence and diversity. This is an appropriate government role and requires a more aggressive approach than is visible at present.

As a related issue, ONC's current approach has the effect of postponing the development of a genuinely universal "syntax" (that is, the formatting of data that are exchanged and the details of exchange protocols) until after the government has harmonized the "semantics" (that is, the clinical or operational *meaning* of the data, or its human understanding) from many different health IT-related realms. This approach implies a focus on achieving some harmonization between taxonomies for diagnosis, for test results, for genetic information, for billing codes, for the particulars of medical instrumentation, and so forth. We urge reconsideration of this approach.

A large body of experience in other domains suggests that creative and entrepreneurial energies are best unleashed by standardizing a syntax that is broadly extensible into different semantic spaces. A much-studied historical example[86] is the language XML ("extensible markup language") and its many off-shoots. If an XML-like universal exchange language for health IT were even minimally standardized, then many existing semantic taxonomies could immediately be mapped to it. Would these be instantaneously harmonized? No. But there would be immediate market incentives toward harmonization, because vendors could compete on how broadly their products "understand" the existing semantic spaces. Rather than a never-ending, Sisyphean government approach to harmonization, the existence of an extensible standardized syntax would promote a market-driven, largely nongovernment, ongoing process. This is a case where government needs to define a (syntax-based) approach that opens the market to new players, and then largely get out of the way.

As mentioned, ONC's CDA is a foundational step in the right direction. However, the thrust of CDA seems largely that it be an extensible wrapper that can hold a variety of structured reports or documents, each with vocabulary-controlled metadata. While this shares many features with the universal exchange language that we envisage, it lacks many others. In particular, it perpetuates the record-centric notion that data elements should "live" inside documents (albeit metadata tagged). We think that a universal exchange language must facilitate the exchange of metadata tagged elements at a more atomic and disaggregated level, so that their varied assembly into documents or reports can itself be a robust, entrepreneurial marketplace of applications. In a similar vein, we view the semantics of metadata tags as an arena in which new players can participate (by "publishing"), not as one limited to a vocabulary controlled by the government.

ONC's cautious approach on these two issues is understandable: the problem itself is inherently complex, and the Office is under pressure from parties who would like the bar for receiving payments under ARRA to be set low. However, we are concerned that this direction, pace, and actions are not currently sufficient to achieve, in the necessary time frame, the President's goal that the Nation have a health IT system adequate to support efforts to increase the quality and decrease the cost of healthcare. Some additional guidance for ONC relates to its support of CMS and is discussed in the next section.

Guidance on Meaningful Use Requirements

Earlier we discussed the broad discretionary powers given to CMS, under ARRA, to define what constitutes meaningful use of EHR technology. In Chapters 4 and 5, we outlined a vision of what ought to be achievable, over the mid- and long-term, as a state-of-the-art national health IT infrastructure. Here, we put these pieces together to suggest what CMS should be doing now.

To accelerate the adoption of a universal exchange language, HHS should specify that meaningful use measures reported to CMS be captured in a tagged data element format.[87] To meet these criteria in the short term, some healthcare providers with legacy EHR systems would probably add middleware to extract and operate on data-level clinical information. Large vendors of EHR systems would likely offer upgrades to meet the CMS requirements.

Such a meaningful use data policy would accomplish several things. First, it would advance EHR technologies in the direction of being able to generate data needed to support other aspects of meaningful use, for example, advanced clinical decision support. Second, this substrate of data will catalyze a host of new IT applications for physicians and hospitals to improve the quality and efficiency of care. Third, this policy eliminates the incentive for vendors to "hard wire" into EHRs the specific quality measures currently required to qualify for meaningful use, instead motivating them to provide a flexible framework into which specified reporting items can be easily inserted. This is important because meaningful use measures will change over time as the art and science of quality measurement improve and as more clinically meaningful measurement constructs become available. If providers are required to pay for expensive system upgrades as new measures are implemented, their support for both the technology and for quality assurance programs will quickly dissipate. Moreover, providers need flexibility in their EHRs to respond to the unique quality-reporting requirements of different health plans and to satisfy licensure, certification, and accrediting organizations with the least possible added burden.

To support this type of meaningful use policy, ONC should issue reference standards with which EHR, software, and middleware vendors would need to comply. The original set of standards for EHR certification[88] implementing HITECH relies heavily on existing standards for the interoperability of health information technologies, including those established and/or promoted by the Health Level 7 standards organization (HL7), NIST, and Integrating the Healthcare Enterprise (IHE). These standards were chosen in an attempt to provide a "minimum set of transport, content, and vocabulary standards required to drive or enhance the predictability of data exchange when used in EHR technologies, in order to drive adoption". We would like to see ONC focus on enabling and accelerating health information exchange at the level of the datum, rather than the message or document, while developing a corresponding reference implementation to verify interoperability. This conceptually straightforward approach to certification would allow flexibility and continued innovation in quality measurement and reporting without adding an extra administrative burden.

For its part, CMS's approach to innovation in quality assessment will need major structural and technical overhauls, and to share the visionary and strategic goals of ONC and the President, so that it advances the state of the art in both clinical practice and health IT. Now, for Stage 1 of meaningful use, CMS will require a set of objectives/measures for eligible professionals and 23 for hospitals. In selecting clinical quality measures for physicians, CMS chose to use a subset of measures from its Physician Quality Reporting Initiative. These measures are highly specified and can be submitted to (and received by) CMS only through specific, limited, technical methods.

PCAST has two concerns with this approach. The first concern is that although isolated, condition-specific measures such as "percent of patients with blood pressure under control" are relevant to population health, they are not adequate to assess the broad range of competencies required for physicians and healthcare organizations to deliver safe and effective care. There is good evidence that real improvements in quality will result only from generating and acting on data that reflect the multidimensional aspects of the clinical practice.[89] Today, large integrated group practices can often generate more sophisticated quality metrics and feedback to physicians than what CMS plans to require. It would be unfortunate if CMS were to re-focus these organizations on less effective measures. As another example, some medical specialty boards and health plans are creating comprehensive assessments of a physician's skills in a particular clinical area.[90] These assessments might combine clinical data elements from a physician's practice with results from a test of knowledge, a review of clinical practice systems, and patient experience surveys, all while testing the psychometric properties of new or different combinations of these various data elements. Such innovation in quality measurement and feedback should lead to innovation in practice improvement cycles comparable to other modern engineering standards.[91] CMS should develop a roadmap for expanding its quality measures to reflect improvements in both information technology and methods of quality assessment.

Our second concern is that clinical quality reporting to CMS is limited to the technical specifications of a single designated consensus body, the National Quality Forum (NQF). This in turn limits both the scope of kinds of measures and the technical specifications that CMS is able and willing to accept. The law contains language allowing an alternate pathway for measures if justified by the Secretary of HHS, but that pathway has not been used. We think that wider use of this alternate pathway provision would allow for more innovation and more meaningful quality assessment than is possible using only computable data that have been electronically "defined" for some other purpose. Moving to a tagged data element environment would allow much greater flexibility of quality assessments. It also would require improvement in CMS's ability to receive more complex data as described above. With new resources and the charge from the PPACA, CMS should ensure that this flexibility is built into its future rulemaking.

CMS's attempt to synergize the *Physician Quality Reporting Initiative* and meaningful use programs and reduce the reporting burden on physicians is a very reasonable approach during the first years of implementation, and is required by legislation. Going forward, however, quality improvement information will be richer, more secure, and timelier if gathered and delivered through Internet-accessible systems.

CMS needs to take specific actions that will demonstrate the value of tagged data element exchange. Adjusting fee-for-service payments based on currently reportable quality measures may spur at least some providers to become more sophisticated users of health IT. But it will not bring healthcare closer to the vision described in Chapter Two if the goal is only to achieve higher scores on specific measures. In Chapter Six, we discussed how CMS demonstrations projects such as the primary care medical home and accountable care organization models would shift the payment focus toward coordinated, integrated care. These models are potentially highly complementary to investments in health IT. CMS could further this connection and perhaps make these models more likely to succeed by requiring that demonstration sites have EHR technologies capable of more than reporting specified measures. These capabilities should include delivering and retrieving metadata-tagged, patient-centered, and patient-authorized information with other networks and sources such as PHRs and public health data aggregators. In addition, it will be important for CMS to document and publicly share what is learned about the contributions of such exchanges to the effectiveness of these new models and the results they achieve.

CMS needs a more aggressive program to support the growth of clinical decision support and secondary data uses. Chapter Three discussed the many problems with the "usability" of EHRs from the clinician's perspective. Most of today's systems do not format information in such a way that it reflects the decision-making and information-flow processes of medical care. Instead, their information display is codified in a series of "pages" that can hamper care while providers work through an electronic version of their written record. Software is needed that is more flexible and can deliver the relevant data that the physician and patient require at the point of care, including the ability to intelligently retrieve information for advanced clinical decision support (such as evidence-based guidelines, genetic information, and clinical trial results).

Federal policies also could seed the development of applications that can improve the capabilities of Federal and public health agencies to leverage large stores of electronic data to advance national health system objectives. Specifically, the Department of Health and Human Services should jumpstart an applications market through both requests for proposals and technology transfer agreements for the secondary use of EHR data. This market could result in the development of a very wide range of applications, including software to support pilot projects for benchmarking, coordination of new ONC objectives toward tagged data element ecosystems with entities developing adverse event and syndromic surveillance networks, tools and training to enable the gathering and input of research-quality data within a fully functional EHR, and the development of a test network for comparative effectiveness research.

Finally, we return to the serious challenge posed by CMS's antiquated IT infrastructure, and the pressing need for its modernization, as has already been recognized by CMS leadership. CMS needs to ensure that it does not replace one inflexible architecture with another. While it is outside of our charge to anticipate the conclusions of a recently initiated National Research Council study of CMS information system capability, we would be surprised if a modern solution did not include most of the following elements: (1) a hardware infrastructure based on continuously upgradeable commodity data center technology; (2) a distributed, redundant, reliable storage system that logically presents as a unified, global file system; (3) a software infrastructure based on standard tools and APIs for distributed computing; (4) data consistency maintained by well-understood distributed transaction management protocols; (5) a well-specified protocol stack (most likely with remote procedure calls on top of TCP) and carefully specified interface formats. As discussed in Chapter Three, Federal IT projects of this magnitude frequently incur cost overruns and schedule slippages, and can take many years to complete. Rapid and otherwise achievable progress in health IT, as envisioned by ONC and (even more aggressively) by this report, could be forestalled or derailed if it becomes tied to CMS's formidable IT challenges.

IX. Recommendations

A number of specific recommendations for the short- and mid-term follow from the discussions contained in this report.

The Chief Technology Officer of the United States should:

- In coordination with the Office of Management and Budget (OMB) and the Secretary of HHS, and using technical expertise within ONC, develop within 12 months a set of metrics that measure progress toward an operational, universal, national health IT infrastructure. Research, prototype, and pilot efforts should not be included in this metric of operational progress.
- Annually, assess the Nation's progress in health IT by the metrics developed, and make recommendations to OMB and the Secretary of HHS on how to make more rapid progress.

The Office of the National Coordinator should:

- Move more boldly to ensure that the Nation has electronic health systems that are able to exchange health data in a universal manner based on metadata-tagged data elements. In particular, ONC should signal now that systems will need to have this capability by 2013 in order to be deemed as making “meaningful use” of electronic health information under the HITECH Act.
- Act to establish initial minimal standards for the metadata associated with tagged data elements, and develop a roadmap for more complete standards over time.
- Facilitate the rapid mapping of existing semantic taxonomies into tagged data elements, while continuing to encourage the longer-term harmonization of these taxonomies by vendors and other stakeholders.
- Support the development of reference implementations for the use of tagged data elements in products. Certification of individual products should focus on interoperability with the reference implementations.
- Set standards for the necessary data element access services (specifically, indexing and access control) and formulate a strategic plan for bringing such services into operation in an interoperable and intercommunicating manner. Immediate priority should be given to those services needed to locate data relating to an individual patient.
- Facilitate, with the Small Business Administration, the emergence of competitive companies that would provide small or under-resourced physician practices, community-based long-term care facilities, and hospitals with a range of cloud-based services.
- Ensure that research funded through the SHARP (Strategic Health IT Advanced Research Projects) program on data security include the use of metadata to enable data security.

The Centers for Medicare & Medicaid Services should:

- Redirect the focus of meaningful use measures as rapidly as possible from data collection of specified lists of health measures to higher levels of data exchange and the increased use of clinical decision supports.
- Direct its efforts under the Patient Protection and Affordable Care Act toward the ability to receive and use data from multiple sources and formats.
- In parallel with (i.e., without waiting for) the NRC study on IT modernization, begin to develop options for the modernization and full integration of its information systems platforms using modern technologies, and with the necessary transparency to build confidence with Congress and other stakeholders.
- When informed by the preliminary and final NRC study reports, move rapidly to implement one or more of the options already formulated, or formulate new options as appropriate, with the goal of making substantial progress by 2013 and completing implementation by 2014. CMS must transition into a modern information technology organization, allowing integration of multiple components and consistent use of standards and processes across all the provider sectors and programs it manages.

- Exercise its influence as the Nation's largest healthcare payer to accelerate the implementation of health information exchange using tagged data elements. By 2013, meaningful use criteria should include data submitted through reference implementation processes, either directly to CMS or (if CMS modernization is not sufficiently advanced) through private entities authorized to serve this purpose.
- By 2013, provide incentives for hospitals and eligible professionals to submit meaningful use clinical measures that are calculated from computable data. By 2015, encourage or require that quality measures under all of its reporting programs (the Physician Quality Reporting Initiative, hospitals, Medicare Advantage plans, nursing homes, etc.) be able to be collected in a tagged data element model.

The Department of Health and Human Services should:

- Develop a strategic plan for rapid action that integrates and aligns information systems through the government's public health agencies (including FDA, CDC, NIH, and AHRQ) and benefits payment systems (CMS and VA).
- Convene a high-level task force to align data standards, and population research data, between private and public sector payers.
- Convene a high-level task force to develop specific recommendations on national standards that enable patient access, data exchange, and de-identified data aggregation for research purposes, in a model based on tagged data elements that embed privacy rules, policies and applicable patient preferences in the metadata traveling with each data element.

IX. Recommendations

- As the necessary counterpart to technical security measures, propose an appropriate structure of administrative, civil, and criminal penalties for the misuse of a national health IT infrastructure and individual patient records, wherever such data may reside.
- Appoint a working group of diverse expert stakeholders to develop policies and standards for the appropriate secondary uses of healthcare data. This could be tasked to the Interagency Coordinating Council for Comparative Effectiveness Research.
- With FDA, bring about the creation of a trusted third-party notification service that would identify and implement methods for re-identification of individuals when data analysis produces important new findings.

Other or multiple agencies:

- AHRQ should be funded to develop a test network for comparative effectiveness research. The FDA, and also other HHS public health agencies, should enable medical researchers to gain access to de-identified, aggregated, near-real-time medical data by using data element access services.

- HHS should coordinate ONC activities with CDC, FDA, and any other entities developing adverse event and syndromic surveillance networks.
- The Department of Defense and the Department of Veteran Affairs should engage with ONC and help to drive the development of standards for universal data exchange of which they can become early adopters.

APPENDIX A: EXPERT INPUT

Expert Input into Health Information Technology Report. PCAST is grateful for the input of these individual experts. Listing here does not imply endorsement of this report or its recommendations.

Jonathan Bush
Chief Executive Officer
Athenahealth

David Blumenthal
National Coordinator
Office of the National Coordinator for
Health Information Technology
Department of Health and Human Services

Julie Boughn
Director and Chief Information Officer, Office of
Information Services
Centers for Medicare & Medicaid Services

Aneesh Chopra
Chief Technology Officer
Associate Director for Technology
Office of Science and Technology Policy

Janet Corrigan
President and Chief Executive Officer
The National Quality Forum

Peter Cullen
Chief Privacy Strategist Microsoft Corp.

Nancy-Ann DeParle
Director, White House Office of Health Reform

Mary Durham
Senior Investigator
Director, Center for Health Research
Vice President for Research
Kaiser Foundation Hospitals

Spike Duzor
Director, Division of Survey Management & Data Release
Centers for Medicare & Medicaid Services

Carl Dvorak
Executive Vice President Epic

Sean Eddy
Group Leader
HHMI Janelia Farm Research Campus

Colin Evans
President and Chief Executive Officer Dossia

Craig Feied
Professor of Emergency Medicine at Georgetown University
Chief Health Strategy Officer, Microsoft Corp.

Douglas Fridsma
Acting Director, Office of Interoperability and Standards
Office of the National Coordinator for
Health Information Technology
Department of Health and Human Services

Charles Friedman
Chief Scientific Officer
Office of the National Coordinator for Health Information Technology
Department of Health and Human Services

John Glaser
Senior Advisor
Office of the National Coordinator for
Health Information Technology
Department of Health and Human Services

Arthur Glasgow
Senior Vice President and General Manager of
Health Information Networks
Ingenix

Richard Hodes
Director
National Institute on Aging
U.S. National Institutes of Health

Marjorie Kanof
Managing Director, Health Care
Government Accountability Office

Martha Kelly
Assistant Director, Health Care
Government Accountability Office

Carl Kesselman
Professor of Industrial and Systems Engineering
Fellow in the Information Sciences Institute
Viterbi School of Engineering
University of Southern California

David Kreiss
Senior Executive Athenahealth

David C. Kibbe
Senior Advisor, American Academy of Family
Physicians
Chair, ASTM International E31Technical
Committee on Healthcare Informatics
Principal, The Kibbe Group LLC

Robert Kocher
Special Assistant to the President for Health Care
National Economic Council

S. Lawrence Kocot
Deputy Director, Engelberg Center for Health
Care Reform
The Brookings Institution

Rebecca Kush
Founder, President, and Chief Executive Officer
Clinical Data Interchange Standards Consortium
(CDISC)

Kipp Lassetter
Chairman and Chief Executive Officer
Medicity
Kenneth Mandl
Associate Professor
Children's Hospital Boston|Harvard Medical
School Harvard-MIT Health Sciences and
Technology

Mark McClellan
Director, Engelberg Center for Health Care
Reform

Leonard D. Schaeffer
Chair in Health Policy Studies
The Brookings Institution

Deven McGraw
Director, Health Privacy Project
Center for Democracy and Technology

Andrew McLaughlin
Deputy Chief Technology Officer
Office of Science and Technology Policy

Farzad Mostashari
Senior Advisor
Office of the National Coordinator for
Health Information Technology
Department of Health and Human Services

Sean Nolan
Chief Architect, Health Solutions Group
Microsoft Corp.

Betty Otter-Nickerson
President Sage
Healthcare Division

Todd Park
Chief Technology Officer
Office of the National Coordinator for
Health Information Technology
Department of Health and Human Services

Daniel Pelino
General Manager, Health Care and Life Sciences
IBM

Richard Platt
Professor and Chair, Harvard Medical School
Department of Population Medicine
Harvard Pilgrim Health Care Institute

Thomas Reilly
Deputy Director, Office of Research,
Development, and Information
Centers for Medicare & Medicaid Services

Andrew Slavitt
Chief Executive Officer
Ingenix

Jean Slutsky
Director, Center for Outcomes and Evidence
Agency for Healthcare Research and Quality
U.S. Department of Health and Human Services

Barry Straub
Chief Medical Officer
Centers for Medicare & Medicaid Services

Marilyn Tavenner
Principal Deputy and Chief Operating Officer
Centers for Medicare & Medicaid Services

Tony Trenkle
Office of E-Health Standards & Services
Centers for Medicare & Medicaid Services

Adindu Uzoma
Senior Fellow and Chief Scientist Ingenix

Thomas Valuck
Senior Vice President, Strategic Partnerships
National Quality Forum

Janet Woodcock
Director, Center for Drug Evaluation and Research
U.S. Food and Drug Administration

APPENDIX B: ACKNOWLEDGMENTS

Joe Alper Writer

Aman Bhandari
Policy Analyst
Office of Science and Technology Policy

Kathleen Black
Intern
Office of Science and Technology Policy

Judith Hautala
Core Research Staff Member, Life Sciences
Science Technology Policy Institute

Peter Haynes
Senior Director, Advanced Strategies and Research
Microsoft Corp.

Steve Olson
Writer

Christina Viola Srivastava
Research Associate
Science Technology Policy Institute

Mark Shankar
Intern
Office of Science and Technology Policy

Leslie Tucker
Policy Director
American Board of Internal Medicine

APPENDIX C: GLOSSARY

Anonymize–Removing all personal identifiers from data

Authentication–Determining the identity of a principal

Authorization–Determining the rights of an authenticated principal

Clinical decision support–Bringing relevant information to the clinician, at the right time and place, to enable optimal health care

Cloud-based–A technology that allows software to be run and data to be stored on remote servers

Comparative effectiveness research–Research that informs clinical decisions by comparing evidence on the benefits, harms, and effectiveness of different treatments

Data element access services–Services that are associated with crawling, indexing, security, identity, authentication, authorization, and privacy

Data-centric–A focus on the specific data relevant to a given task

Data element indexing–Process and infrastructure for locating data elements, similar to today's web search engines

De-identified–Data with all patient identifying information removed, but with the possibility of providing information back to the patient under specified circumstances

Digital signature–Cryptographic method for ensuring that data cannot be altered except by the person who created them.

Electronic health record–An electronic record of health-related information for an patient that contains information captured in clinical visits, lab and imaging studies, and other information important to the patient's medical past

Encryption–Technology of making data completely unreadable except by a person in possession of the corresponding "key"

Genotype–The genetic makeup of a specific human being

Health information exchange–The mobilization of electronic healthcare information across organizations within a community, region, or hospital system

Health information technology–Technologies that manage and transmit health information for use by providers, consumers, payers, insurers, and all the other pertinent groups

HITECH Act–An act passed by Congress in 2009 that authorizes expenditures of approximately $20 billion over five years to promote the adoption and use of electronic health record technologies that would be connected through a national health information network

Integration engines–An application of a universal exchange language that can facilitate data exchanges with personal health records and other types of EHRs in a cloud

Key–A piece of data that can unlock and make readable cryptographically protected information

Meaningful use–Still pending an official definition from CMS, but ARRA requires that the definition include e-prescribing, the ability to exchange information with other healthcare providers to improve care, and the reporting of clinical quality measures to CMS

Metadata–Information that characterizes data, such as contextual information

Metadata tag–A tag accompanying each piece of data describing the attributes, provenance, and required security protections of that piece of information

Middleware–Software used to extract and reformat data elements from existing clinical systems

Patient-centric–Healthcare organized around the needs, capabilities, and desires of patients, with the goal of optimizing care in part through greatly improved uses of data

Personal health record–An electronic record of health information that is maintained, controlled, and shared by a patient-consumer

Personalization–Tailoring medical care to be optimized for the unique individual characteristics of the particular patient

Physician Quality Reporting Initiative–Established under the 2006 Tax Relief and Health Care Act, the initiative provides physicians with a financial incentive to voluntarily provide CMS with a report on three or more chosen quality measures that applies to their Medicare patient base

Post-marketing surveillance–A system by which to identify adverse events that did not appear during the drug approval process

Primary care medical home–A model of care that places the patient and primary care physician at the center of a virtual organization that is paid a fee to coordinate all care the patient receives from specialists and other providers

Randomized clinical trials–A type of clinical trial in which participants are randomly assigned to different forms of treatment

Semantics–The clinical or operational meaning of data

Service-oriented architecture–An approach to health IT that involves using software policies, practices, and frameworks to enable one user to access sets of "services" on another party's computers and data

Standardized health records–Health records that follow a standardized format that is comparable to all other formats and can be accessed by all necessary parties

Syndromic surveillance–Surveillance using health-related data that precedes diagnosis and signals a sufficient probability of a case or an outbreak to warrant a further public health response

Syntax–The formatting of data that are exchanged, as well as the details of the exchange protocols, including privacy protection and other important aspects

Appendix C: Glossary

Tagged data elements–Data accompanied by metadata describing the attributes and privacy protections of the data

Two-factor authentication–The use of two of the following three in determining the identify of a principal: physical credentials (such as smartcards), biometrics (such as fingerprints), and a secret (such as a password)

Universal exchange language–A common language and format in which all electronic health systems can exchange data

Usability–The ease with which physicians and other healthcare providers can learn to use electronic records, capture data from clinical encounters, and then make use of the data to improve care delivery

Value-based purchasing–The concept that buyers should hold providers of health care accountable for both the cost and quality of care

VistA–An integrated system of software applications that directly supports patient care at Veterans Health Administration facilities

XML–Also known as extensible markup language, a set of rules for encoding documents in machine-readable form

APPENDIX D: ABBREVIATIONS

ACO	Accountable Care Organization
AHRQ	Agency for Health Care Research and Quality
ARRA	American Recovery and Reinvestment Act
CDA	Clinical Document Architecture
CDC	Centers for Disease Control & Prevention
CDS	Clinical Decision Support
CMS	Centers for Medicare & Medicaid Services
EHR	Electronic Health Record
FDA	Food and Drug Administration
HIE	Health Information Exchange
HHS	U.S. Department of Health and Human Services
HIPAA	Health Insurance Portability and Accountability Act
HL7	Health Level 7, Inc.
IHE	Integrating the Healthcare Enterprise
IOM	Institute of Medicine
ONC	Office of the National Coordinator
NHIN	Nationwide Health Information Network
NIST	National Institute of Standards and Technology
PCIP	Primary Care Information Project
PCMH	Primary Care Medical Home
PHR	Personal Health Record
PPACA	Patient Protection and Affordable Care Act
RHIO	Regional Health Information Organizations
SHARP	Strategic Health IT Advanced Research Projects
VHA	Veterans Health Administration

End Notes

[1] Network effect is defined as the user externality by which the more people who use a network, the greater its value to each of them. The classic example is the rapid adoption of universal telephone service in the early 20th Century.

[2] Dr. Varmus resigned from PCAST on July 9, 2010 and subsequently became Director of the National Cancer Institute (NCI).

[3] Agency for Healthcare Research and Quality. 2010. Health Care Costs Fact Sheet. See www.ahrq.gov/news/costsfact.htm

[4] Anderson, G., and P. Markovich. 2009. *Multinational Comparisons of Health Systems Data, 2009*. New York: The Commonwealth Fund.

[5] Terms in bold-faced type the first time they appear in this report are defined in the glossary.

[6] Chaudhry, B., J. Wang, S. Wu, M. Maglione, W. Mojica, E. Roth, S. C. Morton, and P. G. Shekelle. 2006. Systematic review: impact of health information technology on quality, efficiency, and costs of medical care. *Annals of Internal Medicine*, 2144:742-752.

[7] Blumenthal, D. 2010. Launching HITECH. *New England Journal of Medicine,* 362:382-385.

[8] National Center for Health Statistics. December 2009. Electronic Medical Record/Electronic Health Record Use by Office-based Physicians: United States, 2008 and Preliminary 2009.

[9] The working group members are listed in page 7.

[10] P.L. 111-5, "American Recovery and Reinvestment Act of 2009" (ARRA), 111 th Congress.

[11] Foreshadowing discussion later in this report, a more technical description of the common framework is: (1) a universal extensible language for the exchange of health information based on "metadata-tagged data elements," (2) a standard for a minimal set of metadata that specifically enforce privacy safeguards on each individual piece of data, and (3) the development of a secure national infrastructure, based on the technology of today's web search engines, for locating and assembling all of a patient's information for clinical encounters and (when de-identified) for public health purposes.

[12] AHRQ web page at http://www.ahrq.gov/about/ataglance.htm

[13] Healthcare IT News (February 26, 2010) at http://www.healthcareitnews.com/blog/should-fda-regulate-ehr-safety

[14] Brownstein, J. S., C. Clark, B. S. Freifeld, E. H. Chan, M. Keller, A. L. Sonricker, S. R. Mekaru, and D. L. Buckeridge. 2010. Information Technology and Global Surveillance of Cases of 2009 H1N1 Influenza. *New England Journal of Medicine,* 362:1731-1735.

[15] For example, given an entry containing a laboratory test result, one might deduce the name of the physician who ordered the test from a case note with a corresponding date (context present, but implicit); but, for the case of an equipment recall, one might not at all be able to deduce the brand of medical equipment used (missing context).

[16] Provenance includes information about the data's source and the processing that the data have undergone.

[17] Brynjolfsson, E, and L. M. Hitt. 1998. Beyond the Productivity Paradox: Computers are the Catalyst for Bigger Changes. See http://ebusiness.mit.edu/erik/bpp.pdf

[18] E.g., Garwin, R. L. 1968. Impact of Information-Handling Systems on Quality and Access to Health Care. *Public Health Reports*, 83(5):346-351.

[19] See http://www.cdc.gov/nchs/data/hestat/emr_ehr/emr_ehr.htm Primary care physicians and those practicing in large groups, hospitals or medical centers, and the western region of the United States were more likely to use electronic health records.

[20] A growing literature demonstrates a positive return on investment for EHRs in small practices, but the larger part of the benefit is not captured.

[21] Stead, W. W., and H. S. Lin, Eds. 2009. Computational Technology for Effective Health Care: Immediate Steps and Strategic Directions. Washington, DC: National Academies Press. http://www.nap.edu/catalog.php?record_id=12572

[22] Schiff, G. D, and D. W. Bates. 2010. Can Electronic Clinical Documentation Help Prevent Diagnostic Errors? *New England Journal of Medicine,* 362:1066-1069.

[23] Nass, S. J., L. A. Levit, and L. O. Gostin, Eds. 2009. Beyond the HIPAA Privacy Rule: Advancing Research, Improving Health Through Research. Washington, DC: National Academy Press. http://www.nap.edu/catalog.php?record_id=12458

[24] Asch, S. M., et al. 2004. Comparison of Quality of Care for Patients in the Veterans Health Administration and Patients in a National Sample. *Annals of Internal Medicine,* 141:938-945.

[25] VistA: Winner of the 2006 Innovations in American Government Award. 2006. See http://www.innovations.va.gov

[26] VA Receives 2006 Innovations in Government Award. 2006. See http://www1.va.gov/opa/pressrel/pressrelease.cfm?id=1152

[27] VistA: Winner of the 2006 Innovations in American Government Award. 2006. See http://www.innovations.va.gov

[28] R. Kahn. 2010. Kaiser Permanente Completes Electronic Health Record Implementation. Available at http://xnet.kp.org/newscenter/pressreleases/nat/2010/030310ehrcomplete.html

[29] Fast Facts about Kaiser Permanente. Available at http://xnet.kp.org/newscenter/aboutkp/fastfacts.html

[30] Weissberg, J. Perspective: Electronic Health Records in a Large, Integrated Health System: It's Automatic....NOT! At Least, Not Yet. National Quality Measures Clearinghouse.

[31] Kweder S. 2004. Vioxx and Drug Safety. Available at http://www.fda.gov/NewsEvents/Testimony/ucm113235.htm

[32] Chen, C., T. Garrido, D. Chock, G. Okawa, and L. Liang. 2009. The Kaiser Permanente Electronic Health Record: Transforming and Streamlining Modalities Of Care. *Health Affairs,* 28: 323-333.

[33] Ibid.

[34] "Sutter Health and Affiliated Palo Alto Medical Foundation Praised by U.S. Health and Human Services for IT Innovation." 2005. See http://www.sutterhealth.org/about/news/news_pamf-ehr.html

[35] Academy Health. "HIT and HSR for Actionable Knowledge: Description of Partnering Health Systems. Partner: Geisinger Health System." See http://www.academyhealth.org/files/HIT/Geisinger%20Health%20System_1wfs.pdf

[36] Pham, H. H., D. Schrag, A. S. O'Malley, B. Wu B, and P. B. Bach. 2007. Care Patterns in Medicare and Their Implications for Pay for Performance. *New England Journal of Medicine,* 356(11):1130-1139.

[37] Robert Wood Johnson Foundation. Aligning Forces for Quality. See http://www.forces4quality.org/welcome

[38] GAO. 2009. "Social Security Administration: Effective Information Technology Management Essential for Data Center Initiative," GAO-09-662T.

[39] See, for example, GAO, 2008, "Information Technology: Agencies Need to Establish Comprehensive Policies to Address Changes to Projects' Cost, Schedule, and Performance Goals," GAO-08-925; GAO, 2008, "DOD Business Systems Modernization: Progress in Establishing Corporate Management Controls Needs to Be Replicated Within Military Departments," GAO-08-705; and GAO, 2008, "Environmental Satellites: Polar-Orbiting Satellite Acquisition Faces Delays, Decisions Needed on Whether and How to Ensure Climate Data Continuity," GAO-08-518.

[40] Elm, J.P., Goldenson, D., El Emam, K., Donitelli, N., and Neisa, A. 2008. Survey of Systems Engineering Effectiveness—Initial Results. Carnegie Mellon University/SEI, CMU/SEI-2008-SR-034, at http://www.sei.cmu.edu/library/abstracts/reports/08sr034.cfm

[41] Kibbe, D. C. 2010. Should Doctors Reject the Government's EHR Incentive Plan? *Family Practice Management,* 17:8.

[42] There are exceptions, however. For example, in Massachusetts, 50% of all providers have comprehensive EHRs, and 33% of all medications are electronically prescribed.

[43] Sprott, D., and L. Wilkes. January 2004. Understanding Service-Oriented Architecture, *Microsoft Architect Journal.*

[44] eHealth Initiative. 2009. Migrating Toward Meaningful Use: The State of Health Information Exchange.

[45] However, a few interesting examples of HIEs working across state boundaries are starting to emerge.

[46] As a privacy choice, a patient might choose to hide even *the existence* of certain data from the DEAS, for example the fact that he/she had received treatment at a particular facility. In making such a choice, the patient would understand that his/her own future physicians would be unaware of this data, with possible negative effect on their ability to deliver the best care.

[47] World Health Organization 2007"Patient Identification", Patient Safety Solutions, vol. 1, solution 2, at http://www.ccforpatientsafety.org/common/pdfs/fpdf/presskit/PS-Solution2.pdf

[48] Markle Foundation 2005 Linking Health Care Information: Proposed Methods for Improving Care and Protecting Privacy, at http://www.connectingforhealth.org/assets

[49] See, e.g., J. Jonas, 2006, Threat and Fraud Intelligence, Las Vegas Style, *IEEE Security and Privacy.*

[50] Government Health IT. June 25, 2010. ONC to issue "rules of the road" for NHIN Exchange. See http://www.govhealthit.com/newsitem.aspx?nid=74064

[51] Currently installed systems that do not encrypt data "at rest" can be upgraded evolutionarily over time, but would be required to encrypt data "in transit" when it is shared with another system.

[52] NPR, Kaiser Foundation, and Harvard School of Public Health. March 2009. Cost, Privacy Top Health Care Concerns.

[53] Electronic Privacy Information Center. Medical privacy public opinion polls.

[54] Lake Research Partners and American Viewpoint. November 2006. Survey Finds Americans Want Electronic Personal Health Information To Improve Own Health Care.

[55] McGraw, D., J. X. Dempsey, L. Harris, and J. Goldman. 2009. Privacy as an Enabler, Not an Impediment: Building Trust into Health Information Exchange. *Health Affairs,* 28(2):416-27.

[56] 45 CFR Parts 160 and 164. Summaries at http://www.hhs.gov/ocr/privacy/hipaa/understanding/index.html

[57] See, for example, Health IT Policy Committee, Privacy and Security Tiger Team, transcript of Consumer Choice Technology Meeting (June 29, 2010), at http://healthit.hhs.gov/portal/server.pt?open=512&mode=2&objID=2833&PageID=19477

[58] The need to have an unbiased second opinion may be an exception to this principle.. Henriksen K. and H. Kaplan, H. 2003. Hindsight bias, outcome knowledge and adaptive learning Quality and Safety in HealthCare 12:ii46-ii50,

[59] Armstrong, D., E. Kline-Rogers, S. M. Jani, et al. 2005. Potential Impact of the HIPAA Privacy Rule on Data Collection in a Registry of Patients with Acute Coronary Syndrome. *Archives of Internal Medicine,* 165:1125-1129.

[60] J.F. Wilson. 2006. Health Insurance Portability and Accountability Act Privacy Rule Causes Ongoing Concerns Among Clinicians and Researchers. Annals of Internal Medicine 145(4):313-316.

[61] Public Law 111-5 (2009), especially Sec. 13405 (42 USC 17935), at http://www.hhs.gov/ocr/privacy/hipaa/understanding/coveredentities/hitechact.pdf#page=39

[62] Nass, S. J., L. A. Levit, and L. O. Gostin, Eds. 2009. Beyond the HIPAA Privacy Rule: Advancing Research, Improving Health Through Research. Washington, DC: National Academy Press. http://www.nap.edu/catalog.php?record_id=12458

[63] But see, for example, PI Newswire, "Medical Records Found in DMV's Dumpster," June 3, 2010, at http://www.pinewswire.net/2010/06/medical

[64] For examples, see "Celebrity Medical Records in Massive UCLA Breach" at http://www.huffingtonpost.com/2008/08/05/celebrity-medical and "Exposed: Clooney's Medical Records" at http://abcnews.go.com/GMA/story?id=3711136&page=1

[65] InformationWeek January 30, 2008. "Laptop Stolen With Personal Data On 300,000 Health Insurance Clients," at http://www.informationweek.com/news/security

[66] WBBM Chicago May 27, 2010. "Nearly 200,000 Are Potential ID Theft Victims," at http://cbs2chicago.com/investigations/ID.theft

[67] While the breach notification requirements of HITECH provide significant incentives for encryption, they do not require it.

[68] Markle Foundation (2006) Implementing a Trusted Information Sharing Environment: Using Immutable Audit Logs to Increase Security, Trust, and Accountability. At http://www.markle.org/downloadable_assets

[69] Abigail has chosen to exclude from indexing, for example, that as a teenager she was once treated for a drug overdose.

[70] Halamka, J. November 11, 2009 *The Magic of Middleware*. Life as a Healthcare CIO, at http://geekdoctor.blogspot.com/2009/11/magic-of-middleware.html

[71] Office of the National Coordinator. May 26, 2010. Beacon Community Program. Available at http://healthit.hhs.gov/portal/server.pt?open=512&objID=1805&parentname=CommunityPage&parentid=2&mode=2&cached=true

[72] Stytz, M., et al. 2010. Electronic Patient Health Record Technology: Status and Challenges. Washington, DC: STPI.

[73] John Halamka, personal communication, based on 2000-2010 Beth Israel Deaconess Medical Center data.

[74] USA Today. October 25, 2009. "R.I. Tracks H1N1 with Electronic Data," at http://www.usatoday.com/news/nation/2009-10-25-rhode-island-flu-tracking_N.htm

[75] Kweder S. November 18, 2004. "Vioxx and Drug Safety." Available at http://www.fda.gov/NewsEvents/Testimony/ucm113235.htm

[76] Nissen, E., and K. Wolski. 2007. Effect of Rosiglitazone on the Risk of Myocardial Infarction and Death from Cardiovascular Causes. *New England Journal of Medicine,* 356(24):2457-2471.

[77] Alliance for Health Reform. March 2006. "Racial and Ethnic Disparities in Health Care." Available at http://www.allhealth.org/publications/pub_38.pdf

[78] The patient Cohen, H., G. Williams, J. Johnson, J. Duan, J. Gobburu, A. Rahman, K. Benson, J. Leighton, S. Kim, R. Wood, M. Rothmann, G. M. Chen, M. Staten, and R. Pazdur. 2002. Approval Aummary for Imatinib Mesylate Capsules in the Treatment of Chronic Myelogenous Leukemia. *Clinical Cancer Research,* 8(5):935-942.

[79] National Cancer Institute. Beta-Carotene Supplements Confirmed as Harmful to Those at Risk for Lung Cancer. Available at http://www.cancer

[80] Gold, T., T. Do T, and W. Dick. 2008. Correlates and Effect of Suboptimal Radiotherapy in Women with Ductal Carcinoma in Situ or Early Invasive Breast Cancer. *Cancer,* 113(11):3108-3115.

[81] W. H. Press. 2009. Bandit Solutions Provide Unified Ethical Models for Randomized Clinical Trials and Comparative Effectiveness Research. *PNAS.* 106:22387-22392.

[82] "Health Level Seven International" at http://www.hl7.org/

[83] World Health Organization. "International Classification of Diseases (ICD)" at http://www.who.int/classifications/icd/en/

[84] The United States Health Information Knowledgebase (USHIK), maintained by AHRQ, maintains metadata on many healthcare-related data standards that could be considered for rapid incorporation. See http://ushik.ahrq.gov/index.html

[85] The crux of the argument in Chapter Six is that this is a public good problem. Market incentives are lacking for private firms to invest in universal exchange capabilities, because they cannot appropriate the benefit.

[86] Gray, J., "A Conversation with Tim Bray." February 16, 2005. http://queue.acm.org/detail.cfm?id=1046941

[87] Although the reported data consists of aggregated counts, not individual patient data, a tagged metadata format can also be applied to this type of data.

[88] Health Information Technology: Initial Set of Standards, Implementation Specifications, and Certification Criteria for Electronic Health Record Technology at http://HealthIT.HHS

[89] Leatherman, S., and A. Epstein. 2010. *Performance Measurement for Health System Improvement.* Cambridge, UK: Cambridge University Press.

[90] Darves, B. June 2008. "Ensuring—and Tracking—Physician Competence." New England Journal of Medicine Career Center. at http://www.nejmjobs.org/career-resources

[91] Gawande, A. 2009. *The Checklist Manifesto: How to Get Things Right.* New York: Metropolitan Books.

In: Transforming Healthcare with Health Information… ISBN: 978-1-61324-417-3
Editors: C. M. Denison, E. L. Montevoy

Chapter 2

THE HEALTH INFORMATION TECHNOLOGY FOR ECONOMIC AND CLINICAL HEALTH (HITECH) ACT*

C. Stephen Redhead

SUMMARY

Lawmakers incorporated the Health Information Technology for Economic and Clinical Health (HITECH) Act as part of the American Recovery and Reinvestment Act of 2009 (H.R. 1), the economic stimulus bill that the President signed into law on February 17, 2009 (P.L. 111-5). The HITECH Act is intended to promote the widespread adoption of health information technology (HIT) to support the electronic sharing of clinical data among hospitals, physicians, and other health care stakeholders. HIT is widely viewed as a necessary and vital component of health care reform. It encompasses interoperable electronic health records (EHRs)—including computerized systems to order tests and medications, and support systems to aid clinical decision making—and the development of a national health information network to permit the secure exchange of electronic health information among providers.

The HITECH Act builds on existing federal efforts to encourage HIT adoption and use. It codifies the Office of the National Coordinator for Health Information Technology (ONCHIT) within the Department of Health and Human Services. ONCHIT was created by Executive Order in 2004 and charged with developing and implementing a strategic plan to guide the nationwide implementation of health information technology (HIT) in the public and private health care sectors. ONCHIT has focused on developing standards necessary to achieve interoperability among varying HIT applications; establishing criteria for certifying that HIT products meet those standards; ensuring the privacy and security of electronic health information; and helping facilitate the creation of prototype health information networks.

The HITECH Act provides financial incentives for HIT use among health care practitioners. It establishes several grant programs to provide funding for investing in HIT infrastructure, purchasing certified EHRs, training, and the dissemination of best practices. It also authorizes grants to states for low-interest loans to help providers finance HIT. Beginning in 2011, the legislation authorizes Medicare incentive payments

* This is an edited, reformatted and augmented version of a Congressional Research Services publication, CRS Report for Congress R40161, from www.crs.gov, dated April 27, 2009.

to encourage doctors and hospitals to adopt and use certified EHRs. Those incentive payments are phased out over time and replaced by financial penalties for physicians and hospitals that are not using certified EHRs. The legislation further authorizes a 100% federal match for payments to certain qualifying Medicaid providers who acquire and use certified EHR technology.

Finally, the HITECH Act includes a series of privacy and security provisions that expand the current requirements under the Health Insurance Portability and Accountability Act (HIPAA). Among other things, the legislation strengthens enforcement of the HIPAA privacy rule and creates a right to be notified in the event of a breach of identifiable health information.

The Congressional Budget Office (CBO) estimates that Medicare and Medicaid spending under the HITECH Act will total $32.7 billion over the 2009-2019 period. CBO anticipates, however, that widespread HIT adoption will reduce total spending on health care. Through 2019, CBO estimates that the HITECH Act will save the Medicare and Medicaid programs a total of about $12.5 billion. Under current law, CBO predicts that about 45% of hospitals and 65% of physicians will have adopted HIT by 2019. CBO estimates that the incentive mechanisms in the HITECH Act will boost those adoption rates to about 70% for hospitals and about 90% for physicians.

INTRODUCTION

The American Recovery and Reinvestment Act of 2009 (ARRA; H.R. 1), which the President signed into law on February 17, 2009 (P.L. 111-5), incorporated the Health Information Technology for Economic and Clinical Health (HITECH) Act. The HITECH Act, based on legislation introduced in the 110th Congress, is intended to promote the widespread adoption of health information technology (HIT) for the electronic sharing of clinical data among hospitals, physicians, and other health care stakeholders.

HIT, which generally refers to the use of computer applications in medical practice, is widely viewed as a necessary and vital component of health care reform. It encompasses interoperable electronic health records (EHRs)—including computerized systems to order tests and medications, and support systems to aid clinical decision making—and the development of a national health information network to permit the secure exchange of electronic health information among providers. The promise of HIT comes not from automating existing practices, but rather as a tool to help overhaul the delivery of care. HIT enables providers to render care more efficiently, for example, by eliminating the use of paper-based records and reducing the duplication of diagnostic tests. It can also improve the quality of care by identifying harmful drug interactions and helping physicians manage patients with multiple conditions. Moreover, the widespread use of HIT would provide large amounts of clinical data for comparative effectiveness research, performance measurement, and other activities aimed at improving health care quality.

Relatively few health care providers have adopted HIT. The most recent estimate suggests that only about 5% of physicians have a fully functional EHR that incorporates all or most of the recommended capabilities, including electronic documentation of physicians' notes, electronic viewing of lab test results and radiological images, electronic prescribing, clinical decision support, and interoperability with other systems.[1] The most important barriers to HIT adoption include the high implementation and maintenance costs, the limited financial incentives for using HIT, and the lack of interoperability.[2]

The HITECH Act includes three sets of provisions to promote HIT adoption. First, it codifies the Office of the National Coordinator for Health Information Technology (ONCHIT) within the Department of Health and Human Services (HHS). Created by Executive Order in 2004, ONCHIT was charged with developing and implementing a strategic plan to guide the nationwide implementation of HIT in the public and private health care sectors. ONCHIT has focused its activities in the following areas: (1) developing vocabulary, messaging, and functional standards necessary to achieve interoperability among varying HIT applications; (2) establishing criteria for certifying that HIT products meet those standards; (3) ensuring the privacy and security of electronic health information; and (4) helping facilitate the creation of prototype health information networks. The goal is to develop a national capability to exchange standards-based health care data in a secure computer environment.

Second, the HITECH Act through a number of mechanisms provides financial incentives for HIT use among health care practitioners. It establishes several grant programs to provide funding for investing in HIT infrastructure, purchasing certified EHRs, training, and the dissemination of best practices. It also authorizes grants to states for low-interest loans to help providers finance HIT. Beginning in 2011, the legislation provides Medicare incentive payments to encourage doctors and hospitals to adopt and use certified EHRs. Those incentive payments are phased out over time and replaced by financial penalties for physicians and hospitals that are not using certified EHRs. In addition to the Medicare incentives, the legislation authorizes a 100% federal match for payments to certain qualifying Medicaid providers for the acquisition and use of certified EHR technology.

Finally, the HITECH Act includes a series of privacy and security provisions that amend and expand the current HIPAA requirements. Among other things, the legislation strengthens enforcement of the HIPAA privacy rule and creates a right to be notified in the event of a breach of identifiable health information.

The Congressional Budget Office (CBO) estimates that the HITECH Act payment incentives (and penalties) will increase spending for the Medicare and Medicaid programs by a total of $32.7 billion over the 2009-2019 period. CBO anticipates, however, that widespread adoption of interoperable EHRs will reduce total spending on health care by decreasing the number of duplicate and inappropriate tests and procedures, reducing paperwork and administrative overhead, and eliminating medical errors. Over the 2009-2019 period, it estimates that the HITECH Act will save the Medicare and Medicaid programs a total of $12.5 billion. When savings to the Federal Employees Health Benefits program and CMS's administrative costs are factored in, CBO estimates overall that the HITECT Act will increase direct federal spending by $20.8 billion.[3] Under current law, CBO predicts that about 45% of hospitals and 65% of physicians will have adopted HIT by 2019. CBO estimates that the incentive mechanisms in the HITECH Act will boost those adoption rates to about 70% for hospitals and about 90% for physicians.

This report provides a summary and explanation of the provisions in the HITECH Act. In order to provide some context for that discussion, the report first gives an overview of prior actions taken by Congress and the Administrations to promote HIT, and briefly describes efforts by the 109th and 110th Congresses to enact comprehensive HIT legislation.

FEDERAL EFFORTS TO PROMOTE HIT

HIPAA Administrative Simplification: Electronic Transactions,Sec urity & Privacy Standards

Congress took an important first step towards promoting HIT when it enacted the Health Insurance Portability and Accountability Act of 1996 (HIPAA; P.L. 104-191). HIPAA imposed new federal requirements on health insurance plans offered by public and private employers, guaranteeing the availability and renewability of health insurance coverage for certain employees and individuals, and limited the use of preexisting condition restrictions. But while HIPAA was primarily concerned with giving consumers greater access to health insurance, the legislation also contained a section, subtitled Administrative Simplification, that included provisions to promote more standardization and efficiency in the health care industry and safeguard personal health information. Under HIPAA Administrative Simplification, the HHS Secretary was required to develop standards to support the growth of electronic record keeping and claims processing in the health care system and to safeguard the privacy of patient records. The standards apply to health care providers (who transmit any health information in electronic form in connection with a HIPAA-specified transaction), heath plans, and health care clearinghouses.

Electronic Transactions and Code Sets

HIPAA instructed the Secretary to issue electronic format and data standards for nine routine administrative and financial transactions between health care providers and health plan/payers. Those transactions include claims and encounter information, payment and remittance advice, and claims status inquiry and response. The electronic transactions standards include several Accredited Standards Committee X12 (ASC X12) standards, as well as a number of code sets (e.g., International Classification of Diseases, 9th Edition, Clinical Modification, or ICD-9CM) used to identify specific diagnoses and clinical procedures that pertain to a patient encounter. HIPAA does not mandate that providers submit transactions electronically, though health plans/payers increasingly require it. However, if a health care provider chooses to submit one or more of the HIPAA-specified transactions electronically, then he or she must comply with the standard for that transaction. In 2001, Congress enacted the Administrative Simplification Compliance (P.L. 107-105), which, among other things, requires Medicare providers to submit claims electronically.

Unique Health Identifiers

HIPAA further required the Secretary to issue national identification numbers for health care providers, health plans, employers, and individuals (i.e., patients) for use in standard transactions. Unique identifiers for providers and employers have been adopted, while the health plan identifier is still under review. The requirement that HHS develop a unique patient identifier has proven too controversial because of privacy concerns and is on hold. Beginning in FY1999, Congress each year has included language in the annual appropriations bill for the Departments of Labor, HHS, and Education prohibiting the use of funds for the development of a unique individual identifier.

Health Information Security

HIPAA's Administrative Simplification provisions also instructed the Secretary to issue security standards to safeguard individually identifiable health information in electronic form against unauthorized access, use, and disclosure. The security rule (45 CFR Parts 160, 164) specifies a series of administrative, technical, and physical security procedures for providers and plans to use to ensure the confidentiality of electronic health information. Administrative safeguards include such functions as assigning or delegating security responsibilities to employees, as well as security training requirements. Physical safeguards are intended to protect electronic systems and data from threats, environmental hazards, and unauthorized access. They include restricting access to computers and off-site backups. Technical safeguards are primarily IT functions used to protect and control access to data. They include using authentication and password controls, and encrypting data for storage and transmission.

The HIPAA security standards are flexible and scalable, allowing covered entities (i.e., health plans, health care providers, and health care clearinghouses) to take into account their size, capabilities, and the costs of specific security measures. The standards are also technology neutral. They do not prescribe the use of specific technologies, so that covered entities will not be bound by particular systems and/or software.

Health Information Privacy

Finally, HIPAA set a three-year deadline for Congress to enact health information privacy legislation. If, as turned out to be the case, lawmakers were unable to pass such legislation before the deadline, the HHS Secretary was instructed to promulgate regulations containing standards to protect the privacy of individually identifiable health information. The HIPAA privacy rule (45 CFR Parts 160, 164) established several individual privacy rights with respect to such protected health information (PHI). First, it established a right of access. Individuals have the right to see and obtain a copy of their own PHI in the form or format they request, provided the information is readily producible in such form or format. If not, then the information must be provided in hard copy or such form or format as agreed to by the covered entity and the individual. The covered entity can impose reasonable, cost-based fees for providing the information. Second, the privacy rule gives individuals the right to amend or supplement their own PHI. Third, individuals have the right to request that a covered entity restrict the use and disclosure of their PHI for the purposes of treatment, payment, or other routine health care operations. However, the covered entity is not required to agree to such a restriction unless it has entered into an agreement to restrict, in which case it must abide by the agreement. Finally, individuals have the right to an accounting of disclosures of their PHI by a covered entity during the previous six years, with certain exceptions. For example, a covered entity is not required to provide an accounting of disclosures that have been made to carry out treatment, payment, and health care operations.

In addition to patient privacy rights, the HIPAA privacy rule placed certain limitations on when and how covered entities may use and disclose PHI. Generally, health plans and health care providers may use and disclose health information for the purpose of treatment, payment, and health care operations without the individual's authorization and with few restrictions. In certain other circumstances (e.g., disclosures to family members and friends), the rule requires plans and providers to give the individual the opportunity to object to the disclosure. The rule also permits the use and disclosure of health information without the individual's permission for various specified activities (e.g., public health oversight, law enforcement) that are not directly connected to the treatment of the individual. For all uses and disclosures of health information that are not otherwise required or permitted by the rule, plans and providers must obtain a patient's written authorization.

The privacy rule incorporates a minimum necessary standard. Whenever a covered entity uses or discloses PHI or requests such information from another covered entity, it must make reasonable efforts to limit the information to the minimum necessary to accomplish the intended purpose of the use or disclosure. There are a number of circumstances in which the minimum necessary standard does not apply; for example, disclosures to or requests by a health care provider for treatment purposes. The rule also permits the disclosure of a "limited data set" for certain specified purposes (e.g., research), pursuant to a data use agreement with the recipient. A limited data set, while not meeting the rule's definition of de-identified information (to which the privacy protections do not apply), has most direct identifiers removed and is considered by HHS to pose a low privacy risk.

Under the HIPAA privacy and security standards, health plans and health care providers may share PHI with their business associates who provide a wide variety of functions for them, including legal, actuarial, accounting, data aggregation, management, administrative, accreditation, and financial services. A covered entity is permitted to disclose health information to a business associate or to allow a business associate to create or receive health information on its behalf, provided the covered entity receives satisfactory assurance in the form of a written contract that the business associate will not use or disclose the information other than as permitted or required by the contract or as required by law, and that the business associate will implement appropriate administrative, technical, and physical safeguards to prevent unauthorized uses and disclosures. Covered entities are not liable for, or required to monitor, the actions of their business associates. If a covered entity finds out about a material breach or violation of the contract by a business associate, it must take reasonable steps to remedy the situation, and, if unsuccessful, terminate the contract. If termination is not feasible, the covered entity must notify HHS.

HIPAA authorized the Secretary to impose civil monetary penalties on any person failing to comply with the privacy and security standards. The maximum civil penalty is $100 per violation and up to $25,000 for all violations of an identical requirement or prohibition during a calendar year. The HHS Office of Civil Rights (OCR) is responsible for enforcing the privacy rule. For certain wrongful disclosures of PHI, OCR may refer the case to the Department of Justice for criminal prosecution. HIPAA's criminal penalties include fines of up to $250,000 and up to 10 years in prison for disclosing or obtaining health information with the intent to sell, transfer or use it for commercial advantage, personal gain, or malicious harm.

Together, the HIPAA privacy and security standards have helped lay the groundwork for the development of a National Health Information Network and the widespread adoption of interoperable EHRs. Information on the HIPAA privacy rule and links to information on the other HIPAA Administrative Simplification standards is at [http://www.hhs.gov/ocr/hipaa].

Medicare Part D: E-Prescribing

Besides HIPAA, the other significant legislative action taken by Congress to promote HIT was the inclusion of electronic prescribing provisions in the Medicare Modernization Act of 2003 (MMA; P.L. 108-173), which created the Part D prescription drug benefit. The MMA established a timetable for the Centers for Medicare and Medicaid Services (CMS) to develop e-prescribing standards, which provide for the transmittal of such information as eligibility and benefits (including formulary drugs), information on the drug being prescribed and other drugs listed in the patient's medication history (including drug-drug interactions), and information on the availability of lower-cost, therapeutically appropriate alternative drugs. CMS issued a set of foundation standards in 2005, then piloted and tested additional standards in 2006. The final Medicare e-prescribing standards, which become effective on April 1, 2009, apply to all Part D sponsors, as well as to prescribers and dispensers that electronically transmit prescriptions and prescription-related information about Part D drugs prescribed for Part D eligible individuals. The MMA did not require Part D drug prescribers and dispensers to e-prescribe. Under its provisions, only those who choose to e-prescribe must comply with the new standards. However, the recently enacted Medicare Improvement for Patients and Providers Act of 2008 (MIPPA; P.L. 110-275) includes an e-prescribing mandate and authorizes incentive bonus payment for e-prescribers between 2009 and 2013. Beginning in 2012, payments would be reduced for those who fail to e-prescribe. Information on the CMS e-prescribing standards is at [http://www.cms.hhs.gov/EPrescribing].

Anti-Kickback Statute, Stark Law

The MMA also instructed the Secretary to establish a safe harbor from penalties under the anti-kickback statute (42 U.S.C. 1320a-7b) and an exception to the Medicare physician self-referral (Stark) law (42 U.S.C. 1395nn) for the provision of HIT and training services used in e-prescribing. The anti-kickback statute prohibits an individual or entity from knowingly or willfully offering or accepting remuneration of any kind to induce a patient referral for, or purchase of, an item or service covered by any federal health care program. The Stark law prohibits physicians from referring patients to any entity for certain health services if the physician (or an immediate family member) has a financial relationship with the entity, and prohibits entities from billing for any services resulting from such referrals, unless an exception applies. Both statutes, which are intended to fight fraud and abuse, are seen as impediments to the dissemination of HIT among health care entities.

In 2006, the Secretary announced final regulations creating new safe harbors and Stark exceptions for certain arrangements involving the donation of electronic prescribing and EHR technologies and training services.[4] That would allow, for example, a hospital to provide such technologies and services to its medical staff, and Medicare Advantage plans to provide such technologies and services to pharmacies and prescribing health care providers.

CMS Grants, Demonstrations and Pay-for-Performance

CMS is administering a number of additional programs to promote HIT adoption. The MMA mandated a three-year pay-for-performance demonstration in four states to encourage physicians to adopt and use HIT to improve the treatment of chronically ill Medicare patients. Physicians participating in the Medicare Care Management Performance (MCMP) demonstration receive bonus payments for reporting clinical quality data and meeting clinical performance standards for treating patients with certain chronic conditions. They are eligible for an additional incentive payment for using a certified EHR and reporting the clinical performance data electronically.

CMS has developed a second demonstration to promote EHR adoption using its Medicare waiver authority. The five-year Medicare EHR demonstration is intended to build on the foundation created by the MCMP program. It will provide financial incentives to as many as 1,200 small- to medium-sized physician practices in 12 communities across the country for using certified EHRs to improve quality, as measured by their performance on specific clinical quality measures. Additional bonus payments will be made based on the number of EHR functionalities a physician group has incorporated into its practice.

The Tax Relief and Health Care Act of 2006 (P.L. 109-432) established a voluntary physician quality reporting system, including an incentive payment for Medicare providers who report data on quality measures. The Medicare Physician Quality Reporting Initiative (PQRI) was expanded by the Medicare, Medicaid, and SCHIP Extension Act of 2007 (P.L. 110-173) and by MIPPA, which authorized the program indefinitely and increased the incentive that eligible physicians can receive for satisfactorily reporting quality measures. In 2009, eligible physicians may earn a bonus payment equivalent to 2.0 percent of their total allowed charges for covered Medicare physician fee schedule services. The PQRI quality measures include a structural measure that conveys whether a physician has and uses an EHR.

The Deficit Reduction Act of 2005 (P.L. 109-171) authorized Medicaid Transformation Grants to states totaling $150 million over two years. The purpose of the grants is to support adoption of innovative methods to improve effectiveness and efficiency in providing medical assistance under Medicaid. In 2007, CMS awarded Medicaid Transformation Grants to 33 states, the District of Columbia, and Puerto Rico. Most of the funds are being used for HIT-related initiatives.

Office of the National Coordinator for Health InformationTechnology

On April 27, 2004, President Bush announced a commitment to the promotion of HIT by calling for the widespread adoption of interoperable EHRs within 10 years. That same day he signed Executive Order 13335 creating ONCHIT to develop, maintain, and direct a strategic plan to guide the nationwide implementation of HIT in the public and private health care sectors. Within three months, ONCHIT published a strategic framework in which it outlined four major goals for HIT: (1) informing clinical practice by accelerating the use of EHRs; (2) interconnecting clinicians allowing them to exchange health information in a secure environment; (3) personalizing health care by enabling consumers to participate more actively in their own care; and (4) improving population health through improved public health surveillance and by accelerating research and its translation into clinical practice.

In fall 2004, ONCHIT solicited public input on a series of questions on whether and how a National Health Information Network should be developed. The questions addressed such topics as organization and business framework, legal and regulatory issues, management and operational considerations, interoperability standards, and privacy and security. Based on the detailed and coordinated responses that it received from a broad array of stakeholders in the health care sector, ONCHIT has undertaken a series of activities to address several important challenges to the nationwide implementation of a HIT infrastructure.

In 2005, the Secretary created the American Health Information Community (AHIC), a public-private advisory body, to make recommendations to the Secretary on how to accelerate the development and adoption of interoperable HIT using a market-driven approach. AHIC and its workgroups have proven to be extremely important in creating a forum to seek input and guidance from a broad range of stakeholders on key HIT issues and policy implications. The AHIC charter required it to provide the Secretary with recommendations to create a successor entity based in the private sector. AHIC Successor, Inc. was established in July 2008 to transition AHIC's accomplishments into a new public-private partnership. That partnership, the National eHealth Collaborative (NeHC), was launched on January 8, 2009.

Developing standards and a process to certify HIT products and services as meeting those standards is a key priority. ONCHIT awarded a contract to the American National Standards Institute (ANSI) to establish a public-private collaborative, known as the Healthcare Information Technology Standards Panel (HITSP), to harmonize existing HIT standards and identify and establish standards to fill gaps. To date, the Secretary has recognized over 100 harmonized standards, including many that need to be used for interoperable EHRs. To ensure that these standards are incorporated into products, a second contract was awarded to the Certification Commission for Healthcare Information Technology (CCHIT), a private, nonprofit organization created by HIT industry associations, which establishes criteria for certifying products that use recognized standards. CCHIT has certified over 150 ambulatory and inpatient EHR products. In August 2006, the President issued Executive Order 13410 committing federal agencies that purchase and deliver health care to require the use of HIT that is based on interoperability standards recognized by the Secretary.

The National Health Information Network (NHIN) is envisioned as a "network of networks"; that is, a nationwide, Internet-based architecture that interconnects state and regional health information exchanges (and other networks). It will be built on a secure platform using a shared set of standards and policies to permit interoperable health information exchange among providers, consumers, and others involved in supporting health care. To facilitate the development of the NHIN, ONCHIT awarded several contracts to develop models of how nationwide electronic health information might work. Each contractor was asked to develop a prototype architecture for the NHIN and to interconnect three communities as a demonstration of the architecture. The initial phase of the project has since been expanded and now involves health information exchanges across the country working cooperatively to identify and implement best practices for health information exchange.

Ensuring the privacy and security of electronic health information is critical to the success of the NHIN and the widespread adoption of interoperable EHRs. ONCHIT has undertaken the development of a national privacy and security framework, using HIPAA as its foundation, to incorporate the needs of health care consumers and build public trust in the new e-health environment. To this end it has awarded a contract to RTI International, which in turn has subcontracted with 33 states and one territory that make up the Health Information Security and Privacy Collaboration (HISPC). HISPC is leveraging input from a broad range of public and private stakeholders in health information exchange to assess the variations in current privacy and security practices and policies. The goal is to identify both best practices and challenges, and develop consensus-based solutions for interoperable electronic health information exchange that protect the privacy and security of health information. Information on ONCHIT's activities and programs is at [http://www.hhs.gov/healthit].

Agency for Healthcare Research and Quality

Within HHS, the Agency for Healthcare Research and Quality (AHRQ) is the principal source of federal HIT grant money. Since 2004, AHRQ has awarded $260 million to support and stimulate investment in HIT. This translates into almost 200 projects in 48 states. AHRQ-funded projects, many of which are focused on rural and underserved populations, cover a broad range of HIT tools and systems, including EHRs, personal health records (PHRs),[5] e-prescribing, privacy and security, quality measurement, and Medicaid technical assistance. In addition, AHRQ created the online National Resource Center for Health IT to disseminate research findings and best practices, facilitate expert and peer-to-peer collaboration, and foster the growth of online communities who are planning to implement HIT. Information on AHRQ's HIT activities and programs is at [http://healthit.ahrq.gov].

Other Federal Agencies

Other federal agencies that purchase health care are also involved in efforts to further the development and broad adoption of HIT. The Department of Defense (DOD), the Department of Veterans Affairs (VA), and the Office of Personnel Management (OPM) have worked with HHS to adopt health information standards for use by all federal health agencies. As part of the Consolidated Health Informatics Initiative, more than 20 federal agencies have agreed to endorse standards that enable information to be shared among agencies and that can serve as a model for the private sector. Over the past few years, OPM has encouraged Federal Employees Health Benefits (FEHB) health benefits plans to increase their use of HIT.

The VA and DOD are both extensive users of HIT. For several years, the VA has used an EHR— the Veterans Health Information Systems and Technology Architecture, or VistA—in providing care to U.S. military veterans. According to the VA, VistA has improved the efficiency of its health care delivery and the quality of the care it provides. DOD has developed and is in the process of implementing an EHR—known as AHLTA (Armed Forces Health Longitudinal Technology Application)—for its health care system. DOD is also working with the VA to develop a way by which health information can be transmitted seamlessly and instantaneously between the two agencies.

HIT Legislation in the 109 and 110 Congresses

109 Congress

The 109th Congress was the first to consider comprehensive HIT legislation. On November 18, 2005, the Senate, by unanimous consent, passed the bipartisan Wired for Health Care Quality Act (S. 1418, S.Rept. 109-111). On July 27, 2006, the House passed the

Health Information Technology Promotion Act (H.R. 4157, H.Rept. 109-603) on a vote of 270-148. The bills, which contained several important differences, were not conferenced. Both bills included comparable provisions establishing ONCHIT, but contained competing language addressing the responsibilities and composition of AHIC and its role in the adoption of interoperability standards. Only the Senate bill addressed certification. S. 1418 also would have authorized grants for health care providers, grants for implementing regional HIT plans, and a state loan program to facilitate HIT adoption. H.R. 4157 included a single HIT grant program for integrated health care systems. Both measures would have authorized a demonstration program, but for differentpurposes. The House measure also included provisions that would have established an anti-kickback safe harbor and Stark exception for the donation of HIT and related support or training services, as well as provisions to expedite updating and modifying the HIPAA electronic transactions and codes standards. The Senate version contained no such provisions.

110 Congress

The Wired for Health Care Quality Act (S. 1693) was reintroduced on June 26, 2007, and ordered reported (as amended) by the Committee on Health, Education, Labor, and Pensions (HELP) on August 1, 2007 (S.Rept. 110-187). In the House, H.R. 6357, the PRO(TECH)T Act of 2008, was introduced by Representatives Dingell and Barton on June 24, 2008, and ordered reported (as amended) by the Committee on Energy and Commerce on September 11, 2008 (H.Rept. 110- 837). No further legislative action was taken on either measure. Like the Senate bill, H.R. 6357 would have codified ONCHIT and authorized grants and loans to promote the adoption of EHRs and the development of health information exchange networks. Unlike S. 1693, however, the House measure also included extensive privacy and security provisions to strengthen the HIPAA rules. A second House bill, H.R. 6898, the Health-e Information Technology Act of 2008, was introduced by Representative Stark on September 15, 2008, and referred to the Committees on Energy and Commerce, Science and Technology, and Ways and Means. Broadly similar to the PRO(TECH)T Act, H.R. 6898 also included Medicare incentive payments to encourage EHR use by hospitals and physicians, as well as financial penalties for providers that failed to adopt HIT.

HITECH Act: Explanation of Provisions

Lawmakers incorporated the HITECH Act in the American Recovery and Reinvestment Act of 2009 (ARRA; H.R. 1, H.Rept. 111-16), the economic stimulus bill that the President signed into law on February 17, 2009 (P.L. 111-5). The HITECH Act is an amalgam of the two House bills from the 110th Congress. It contains three sets of provisions that are expected to boost HIT adoption among health care providers in the coming years. First, it codifies ONCHIT and establishes a process for the development of interoperability standards that support the nationwide electronic exchange of health information among doctors, hospitals, patients, health plans, the federal government, and other health care stakeholders. It also establishes a voluntary certification process for HIT products. The National Institute of

Standards and Technology (NIST) is to provide for the testing of such products to determine if they meet national standards that allow for secure electronic information exchange. After the adoption of an initial set of standards by the end of 2009, the National Coordinator must make an EHR available at a nominal fee, unless it is determined that the needs and demands of providers are being adequately met by the marketplace.

Second, the HITECH Act authorizes funding for several grant programs to support HIT infrastructure, EHR adoption, training, dissemination of best practices, telemedicine, and inclusion of HIT in clinical education. Funds also are provided to states for low-interest loans to help health care practitioners finance HIT. In addition, the legislation provides financial incentives through the Medicare and Medicaid programs to encourage doctors, hospitals, health clinics, and other entities to adopt and use certified EHRs. Medicare incentive payments are phased out over time and replaced with financial penalties for providers that are not using EHRs.

Finally, the HITECH Act expands the HIPAA privacy and security standards. Among other things, it establishes a breach notification requirement for health information that is not encrypted, strengthens enforcement of the HIPAA standards by increasing penalties for violations and provides greater resources for enforcement and oversight activities, places new restrictions on marketing activities by health plans and providers, and creates transparency by allowing patients to request an audit trail showing all disclosures of their electronic health information.

The HITECH Act appears in two separate ARRA titles, each of which is described in the tables below. *Table 1* provides a summary of the HITECH Act provisions in Division A, Title XIII of the economic stimulus bill. Those provisions include ONCHIT and the development and adoption of standards, the grant and loan programs, and the privacy and security requirements. *Table 2* summarizes the HITECH Act's Medicare and Medicaid provisions, which are in Division B, Title IV of the stimulus bill. For each provision, as appropriate, the tables include additional information on existing federal requirements and other relevant administrative activities. Each mention of the Secretary in the tables refers to the Secretary of Health and Human Services. Note: *Table 2* does not include two miscellaneous Medicare provisions added to the HITECH Act, which are unrelated to HIT.[6]

HIT Appropriations in ARR

In addition to the mandatory funding that would become available to health care providers under the HITECH Act's Medicare and Medicaid provisions, the emergency appropriations provisions in ARRA Division A include \$2 billion in discretionary funds for ONCHIT to invest in HIT architecture; provide grants to hospitals, physicians, and other health care providers; and support training programs. In addition, \$85 million is appropriated to the Indian Health Service (IHS) for HIT and telehealth, to be allocated at the discretion of the IHS Director.[7]

Table 1. HITECH Act: Standards Development and Adoption; Grants and Loans; Privacy and Security American Recovery and Reinvestment Act of 2009 (P.L. 111-5): Division A, Title XIII

Topic	Summary of Provision	Current Requirements and Activities
Office of the National Coordinator for Health Information Technology (ONCHIT): Standards Development and Adoption (Subtitle A, Part 1)		
ONCHIT: Purpose and Duties	The Act establishes within HHS the Office of the National Coordinator for Health Information Technology (ONCHIT). The National Coordinator is appointed by the Secretary and report directly to the Secretary. ONCHIT's purpose is to promote the development of a national HIT infrastructure that allows the electronic use and exchange of information, in order to improve health care quality, reduce health care costs and health disparities, improve public health, facilitate research, and promote prevention and management of chronic diseases, among other things. The National Coordinator is charged with the following duties: (1) review and determine whether to endorse standards, implementation specifications, and certification criteria recommended by the HIT Standards Committee (see below); (2) coordinate HIT policy and programs within HHS and with those of other federal agencies and act as a liaison among the HIT Policy and Standards Committees (see below) and the federal government; (3) update and republish the Federal Health IT Strategic Plan (as of June 3, 2008) to include specific objectives, milestones, and metrics with respect to the electronic exchange and use of health information, the utilization of an EHR for each person in the United States by 2014, the incorporation of privacy and security protections for the electronic exchange of an individual's health information, strategies for using HIT to improve health care quality, and plans for ensuring that populations with unique needs, such as children, are appropriately addressed in the technology design, among other things; (4) maintain and update a website to post relevant information about the work related to efforts to promote a nationwide HIT infrastructure; (5) in consultation with the National Institute of Standards and Technology (NIST), keep or recognize a program or programs for the voluntary certification of HIT as being in compliance with applicable certification criteria adopted by the Secretary; (6) prepare several reports, including a report on any additional funding or authority needed to evaluate and develop HIT standards; a report on lessons learned from HIT implementation by major public and private health care systems; a report on the benefits and costs of the electronic use and exchange of health information; an assessment of the impact of HIT on communities with health disparities and in medically underserved areas; and a report estimating the resources needed annually to achieve nationwide adoption of EHRs by 2014, including the resources needed to establish a sufficient HIT workforce; (7) establish a national governance mechanism for the national health information network; and (8) appoint a Chief Privacy Officer of the Office of the National Coordinator to advise the National Coordinator on privacy, security, and data stewardship.	ONCHIT was created by Executive Order 13335, signed by President Bush on April 27, 2004. The National Coordinator was instructed to develop, maintain, and direct a strategic plan to guide the nationwide implementation of interoperable HIT in the public and private health care sectors.

Table 1. (Continued).

Topic	Summary of Provision	Current Requirements and Activities
HIT Policy Committee	The Act establishes an HIT Policy Committee to make policy recommendations to the National Coordinator relating to the implementation of a nationwide HIT infrastructure, including recommending areas in which standards are needed for the electronic exchange and use of health information, and recommending an order of priority for the development of such standards. The Committee is required to provide recommendations in at least the following eight areas: (1) technologies that protect the privacy and security of electronic health information; (2) a nationwide HIT infrastructure that enables electronic information exchange; (3) nationwide adoption of certified EHRs; (4) EHR technologies that allow for an accounting of disclosures; (5) using EHRs to improve health care quality; (6) encryption technologies that render information unusable, unreadable, and indecipherable to unauthorized individuals; (7) the use of electronic systems to collect patient demographic data (consistent with the evaluation of health disparities data under Sec. 1809 of the Social Security Act); and (8) technologies and design features that address the needs of children and other vulnerable populations. The Act describes other areas that the committee might consider, including using HIT to reduce medical errors, and telemedicine. The National Coordinator must take a leading role in the establishment and operations of the HIT Policy Committee. Committee members— appointed by the Secretary, Congress, and the Comptroller General (as specified in the Act)—must represent a balance among various health care sectors so that no one sector unduly influences the Committee's recommendations. The Committee must ensure the participation of outside advisors. The Secretary must publish in the Federal Register and post online all of the Committee's recommendations. The provisions of the Federal Advisory Committee Act (FACA) apply to the HIT Policy Committee.	In 2005, the Secretary created the American Health Information Community (AHIC), a public-private advisory body, to make recommendations to the Secretary on how to accelerate the development and adoption of interoperable HIT using a market-driven approach. The AHIC charter required it to provide the Secretary with recommendations to create a successor entity based in the private se AHIC Successor, Inc. was established in July 2008 to transition AHIC's accomplishments into a new public-private partnership. That partnership, the National eHealth Collaborative (NeHC), was launched on January 8, 2009.
HIT Standards Committee	The Act establishes an HIT Standards Committee to recommend to the National Coordinator standards, implementation specifications, and certification criteria for the electronic exchange of health information. Duties of the HIT Standards Committee include the development, harmonization, and pilot testing of standards, and serving as a forum for the participation of a broad range of stakeholders to provide input on the development, harmonization, and recognition of standards. Not later than 90 days after enactment, the HIT Standards Committee is to outline a schedule (to be updated annually) for assessing the policy recommendations developed by the HIT Policy Committee. In addition, the Committee is to conduct open public meetings and develop a process to allow for public comment on this schedule.	ONCHIT awarded a contract to the American National Standards Institute (ANSI) to establish a public-private collaborative, known as the Healthca Information Technology Standards Panel (HITSP), to harmonize existing HIT standards and identify and has recognized over 100 standards, including many for interoperable EHRs.

Topic	Summary of Provision	Current Requirements and Activities
	The National Coordinator must take a leading role in the establishment and operations of the HIT Standards Committee. Committee members must represent a balance among various health care sectors so that no one sector unduly influences the Committee's recommendations. The Committee must ensure a similar balance in developing procedures for conducting its activities. The Committee must ensure the participation of outside advisors. The Secretary must publish in the Federal Register and post online all of the Committee's recommendations. The provisions of the Federal Advisory Committee Act (FACA) apply to the HIT Standards Committee.	To ensure that these standards are incorporated into products, a second contract was awarded to the Certification Commission for Healthcare Information Technology (CCHIT), a private, nonprofit organization created by HIT industry associations, which establishes criteria for certifying products that use recognized standards. CCHIT has certified over 150 ambulatory and inpatient EHR products.
Adoption of Standards, Implementation Specifications, and Certification Criteria	The Act requires the Secretary, within 90 days of receiving from the National Coordinator a recommendation for HIT standards, implementation specifications, or certification criteria, to determine whether or not to propose adoption of such measures. Adoption is to be accomplished through notice-and-comment rulemaking, whereas a decision not to adopt is to be conveyed in writing to the National Coordinator and the HIT Standards Committee. The Secretary must adopt, through notice-and-comment rulemaking, an initial set of standards by December 31, 2009. The initial standards may be issued as an interim final rule.	
Use of Standards by Private Entities	Nothing in the Act requires (or gives a federal agency new authority to require) a private entity to adopt a standard or implementation specification developed under the Act.	
Federal EHR Technology	The Act requires the National Coordinator to support the development and routine updating of qualified EHR technology and to make such technology available unless the Secretary determines that the needs and demands of providers are being substantially and adequately met through the marketplace. The National Coordinator may charge providers a nominal fee to purchase this technology, taking into account the financial circumstances of smaller and rural providers.	
Open Source HIT Systems	The Act requires the Secretary, in consultation with other federal agencies, to study and report to Congress by October 1, 2010, on the availability and cost of open source HIT systems to federal safety net providers, including smaller and rural providers and those that provide a significant amount of care to the uninsured.	
Transitions	Upon enactment, all functions, personnel, assets, liabilities, and administrative actions of the existing ONCHIT are transferred to the new ONCHIT established by the Act. Nothing in the Act prohibits AHIC Successor, Inc., doing business as the National eHealth Collaborative, from modifying its charter, duties, membership, and any other functions to be consistent with the provisions of this subtitle in a manner that would permit the Secretary to recognize it as the HIT Policy Committee or the HIT Standards Committee.	

Table 1. (Continued).

Topic	Summary of Provision	Current Requirements and Activities
Relations to HIPAA Privacy and Security Rules	The Act specifies that its provisions may not be construed as having any effect on the authorities of the Secretary under HIPAA privacy and security law.	
Application and Use of Adopted Health Information Technology Standards (Subtitle A, Part 2)		
Federal Agencies	The Act requires federal agencies that implement, acquire, or upgrade HIT systems for the electronic exchange of health information to use HIT systems and products that meet the standards adopted by the Secretary under this Act. The President must ensure that federal activities involving the collection and submission of health information are consistent with such standards within three years of their adoption.	In August 2006, President Bush issued Executive Order 13410 committing federal agencies that purchase and deliver health care to require the use of HIT that is based on interoperability standards recognized by the Secretary.
Federal Contractors	The Act requires health care payers and providers that contract with the federal government to use HIT systems and products that meet the standards adopted by the Secretary under this Act.	
Reports	The Act requires the Secretary: (1) within two years and annually thereafter, to report to Congress on efforts to facilitate the adoption of a nationwide system for the electronic exchange of health information; (2) to conduct a study that examines methods to create efficient reimbursement incentives for improving health care quality in federally qualified health centers, rural health clinics and free clinics, and to report to Congress within two years; and (3) to conduct a study of matters relating to the potential use of new aging services technology to assist seniors, individuals with disabilities and their caregivers throughout the aging process, and to report to Congress within two years.	
Testing of Health Information Technology (Subtitle B)		
NIST Testing	The Act requires NIST, in coordination with the HIT Standards Committee, to test HIT standards, as well as support the establishment of a voluntary testing program by accredited testing laboratories.	ONCHIT is working with NIST on testing HIT standards. NIST is assisting with the HITSP standards harmonization process and with CCHIT's certification activities.
Research and Development Programs	The Act requires NIST, in consultation with the National Science Foundation (NSF) and other federal agencies, to award competitive grants to universities (or research consortia) to establish multidisciplinary Centers for Health Care Information Enterprise Integration. The purpose of the Centers is to generate innovative approaches to the development of a fully interoperable national health care infrastructure, as well as to develop and use HIT. The National High-Performance Computing Program must include federal research and development programs related to HIT.	

Topic	Summary of Provision	Current Requirements and Activities
Grant, Loan, and Demonstration Programs (Subtitle C)		
HIT Infrastructure Grants	The Act instructs the Secretary to invest in HIT so as to promote the nationwide use and exchange of electronic health information. The Secretary must invest funds through the different HHS agencies with relevant expertise to support the following: (1) HIT architecture to support the secure electronic exchange of information; (2) EHRs for providers not eligible for HIT incentive payments under Medicare and Medicaid; (3) training and dissemination of information on best practices to integrate HIT into health care delivery; (4) telemedicine; (5) interoperable clinical data repositories; (6) technologies and best practices for protecting health information; and (7) HIT use by public health departments. The Secretary must ensure, to the greatest extent practicable, that funds are used to acquire HIT that meets applicable standards adopted by the Secretary.	Since 2004, AHRQ has awarded $260 million to support and stimulate investment in HIT. AHRQfunded projects, many of which are focused on rural and underserved populations, cover a broad range of HIT tools and systems including EHRs, PHRs, eprescribing, privacy and security, quality measurement, and Medicaid technical assistance. In addition, the Federal Communication Commission's Universal Service Rural Health Care Program has provided $417 million to rural health care providers for telecommunications services, including broadband, to improve health care quality.
HIT Implementation Assistance	The Act requires the National Coordinator, in consultation with NIST, to establish an HIT extension program to assist providers in adopting and using certified HER technology. The Secretary also must create an HIT Research Center to serve as a forum for exchanging knowledge and experience, providing technical assistance to health information networks, and learning about using HIT in medically underserved communities. Finally, the Secretary must fund the creation and operation of HIT Regional Extension Centers, affiliated with nonprofit organizations, to provide assistance to providers in the region. Priority will be given to assisting public, nonprofit, and critical access hospitals, community health centers, individual and small group practices, and entities that serve the uninsured, underinsured, and medically underserved individuals. Regional centers are permitted to receive up to four years of funding, to cover up to 50% of their capital and annual operating and maintenance expenditures. Each center that receives financial support must be evaluated biennially. Within 90 days of enactment, the Secretary must publish in the Federal Register a detailed explanation of the program, procedures to be followed by the applicants, and the maximum support levels expected to be available to centers under the program.	

Table 1. (Continued).

Topic	Summary of Provision	Current Requirements and Activities
State Planning and Implementation Grants	The National Coordinator is authorized to award planning and implementation grants to states or qualified state-designated entities to facilitate and expand electronic health information exchanges. To qualify as a state-designated entity, an entity must be a nonprofit organization with broad stakeholder representation on its governing board and adopt nondiscrimination and conflict-of-interest policies. In order to receive an implementation grant, a state or qualified state-designated entity must submit a plan describing the activities to be carried out to facilitate and expand electronic health information exchange according to nationally recognized standards and implementation specifications. The Secretary annually must evaluate the grant activity under this section and implement the lessons learned from each evaluation in the subsequent round of awards in such a manner as to realize the greatest improvement in health care quality, decrease in costs, and the most effective and secure electronic information exchange. Grants require a match of at least $1 for each $10 of federal funds in FY2011, at least $1 for each $7 of federal funds in FY2012, and at least $1 for each $3 of federal funds in FY2013 and each subsequent fiscal year.	
State Loan Programs	The Act authorizes the National Coordinator to award competitive grants to states or Indian tribes to establish loan programs for health care providers to purchase and upgrade certified EHR technology, train personnel in the use of such technology, and improve the secure electronic exchange of health information. To be eligible, grantees must: (1) establish a qualified HIT loan fund; (2) submit a strategic plan, updated annually, describing the intended uses of the funds and providing assurances that loans will only be given to health care providers that submit required reports on quality measures and use the certified EHR technology supported by the loan for the electronic exchange of health information to improve the quality of care; and (3) provide matching funds of at least $1 for every $5 of federal funding. Loans are repayable over a period of up to 10 years. Each year, the National Coordinator must provide a report to Congress summarizing the annual reports submitted by grantees.Awards are not permitted before January 1, 2010.	
Clinical Education Demonstration	The Act authorizes the Secretary to create a demonstration program for awarding competitive grants to medical, dental, and nursing schools, and to other graduate health education programs to integrate HIT into the clinical education of health care professionals. To be eligible, grantees must submit a strategic plan. A grant may not cover more than 50% of the costs of any activity for which assistance is provided, though the Secretary has the authority to waive that cost-sharing requirement. The Secretary annually must report to designated House and Senate Committees on the demonstrations, with recommendations.	
Medical Informatics Education Grants	The Act requires the Secretary, in consultation with the NSF, to provide financial assistance to universities to establish or expand medical informatics programs.	

Topic	Summary of Provision	Current Requirements and Activities
Reports and Evaluation	The Secretary may require grantees, within one year of receiving an award, to report on the effectiveness of the activities for which the funds were provided and the impact of the project on health care quality and safety. The National Coordinator annually must evaluate the grant activities under this subtitle and implement the lessons learned from each evaluation in the subsequent round of awards in such a manner as to realize the greatest improvement in the quality and efficiency of health care.	
Authorization of Appropriations	The Act authorizes the appropriation of such sums as may be necessary for each of FY2009 through FY2013 to fund the grant, loan, and demonstrations programs.	
HIPAA Privacy and Security Standards (Subtitle D)		
Definitions	The Act defines the following privacy and security terms, in most cases by reference to definitions in the HIPAA Administrative Simplification standards: breach, business associate, covered entity, disclose, electronic health record (EHR), health care operations, health care provider, health plan, National Coordinator, payment, personal health record (PHR), protected health information (PHI), Secretary, security, state, treatment, use, and vendor of personal health records. The term breach means the unauthorized acquisition, access, use, or disclosure of PHI which compromises the security and privacy of such information, but does not include (1) any unintentional acquisition, access, or use of PHI by an individual acting in good faith and under the authority of a covered entity of business, provided the information is not further acquired, used, or disclosed, and (2) any inadvertent disclosure from an individual who is otherwise authorized to access PHI, provided the information received as a result of the disclosure is not further acquired, used, or disclosed without authorization.	
Application of Security Provisions and Penalties to Business Associates	The Act applies the HIPAA security standards and the civil and criminal penalties for violating those standards to business associates in the same manner as they apply to covered entities. It also requires the Secretary, in consultation with industry stakeholders, to issue annual guidance on the most effective and appropriate technical safeguards, including the use of encryption standards recommended by the HIT Policy Committee, for protecting electronic health information.	The HIPAA civil and criminal penalties apply to covered entities. As previously discussed, covered entities are not liable for, or required to monitor, the actions of their business associates. If a covered entity finds out about a material breach or violation of the contract by a business associate, it must take reasonable steps to reme dy the situation, and, if unsuccessful, terminate the contract. If termination is not feasible, the covered entity must notify HHS.

Table 1. (Continued).

Topic	Summary of Provision	Current Requirements and Activities
Notification of Information Breach: HIPAA Covered Entities	In the event of a breach of unsecured PHI that is discovered by a covered entity, the covered entity must notify each individual whose information has been, or is reasonably believed to have been, accessed, acquired, or disclosed as a result of such breach. For a breach of unsecured PHI under the control of a business associate, the business associate upon discovery of the breach must notify the covered entity. All breach notifications have to be made no later than 60 days after their discovery. Notification may be delayed, in the same manner as provided in Section 164.528(a)(2) of the HIPAA privacy rule, if it would impede criminal investigation or damage national security. The provision specifies the methods by which individuals must be notified and the contents of the notification. Notice of the breach must be provided to prominent media outlets serving a particular area if more than 500 individuals in that area are impacted. Covered entities also must immediately notify the Secretary of breaches of unsecured PHI involving 500 or more individuals. If the breach impacts fewer than 500 individuals, the covered entity involved has to maintain a log of such breaches and annually submit it to the Secretary. The Secretary is required to list on the HHS website each covered entity involved in a breach that impacts more than 500 individuals. The Act defines unsecured PHI as information that is not secured through the use of a technology or methodology identified by the Secretary as rendering the information unusable, unreadable, and undecipherable to unauthorized individuals. Within 60 days, and annually thereafter, the Secretary is required to issue guidelines specifying such technologies and methodologies, including the use of encryption standards recommended by the HIT Policy Committee. If the Secretary fails to meet those deadlines, PHI will be considered unsecure if not secured by a technology standard rendering it unusable, unreadable, or indecipherable to unauthorized individuals that was developed or endorsed by a standards development organization accredited by ANSI. The Act requires the Secretary annually to report to Congress on the number and type of breaches, actions taken in response, and recommendations made by the National Coordinator on how to reduce the number of breaches. Within 180 days of enactment, the Secretary is required to issue interim final regulations to implement this section.	The privacy and security rules do not require covered entities to notify HHS or others of a breach of the privacy, security, or integrity of PHI. However, business associate contracts must include a provision requiring business ass covered entities if they become aware of any security incident or any use or disclosure of PHI that is not provided for by the contract.
Privacy Education	The Secretary is required to designate a privacy advisor in each HHS regional office to offer education and guidance to covered entities and business associates. Within 12 months of enactment, OCR must develop and maintain a national education program to educate the public about their privacy rights and the potential uses of their PHI.	The privacy rule requires each covered entity to designate a privacy official for the development and implementation of its policies and procedures.

Topic	Summary of Provision	Current Requirements and Activities
Application of Privacy Provisions and Penalties to Business Associates	Business associates are only permitted to use or disclose PHI if such action is in compliance with the contract. The current provisions regarding a covered entity acting on its knowledge of a material breach or violation by a business associate apply equally to a business associate gaining such knowledge. In the case of a business associate violating the privacy contract requirements in this section, the Act applies the civil and criminal penalties to that business associate in the same manner as they apply to covered entities. Any additional privacy requirements under this subtitle that are made applicable to covered entities also apply to business associates and have to be incorporated into the contract.	The HIPAA civil and criminal penalties apply to covered entities. As previously discussed, covered entities are not liable for, or required to monitor, the actions of their business associates. If a covered entity finds out about a material breach or violation of the contract by a business associate, it must take reasonable steps to remedy the situation, and, if unsuccessful, terminate the contr not feasible, the covered entity must notify HHS.
Patients' Privacy Rights	The Act gives individuals the right to receive an electronic copy of their PHI, if it is maintained in an EHR, and direct the covered entity to transmit such copy to an entity or person clearly designated by the individual. It also requires a health care provider to honor a patient's request that the PHI regarding a specific health care item or service not be disclosed to a health plan for purposes of payment or health care operations, if the patient paid out-of-pocket in full for that item or service. Further, individuals have the right to receive an accounting of PHI disclosures made by covered entities or their business associates for treatment, payment, and health care operations during the previous three years, if the disclosures were through an EHR. Within 6 months of adopting standards on accounting of disclosures, the Secretary must issue regulations on what information shall be collected about each disclosure, taking into account the administrative burden of accounting for such disclosures.	As previously discussed, the privacy rule establishes several federal privacy rights, including the right of access to one's own PHI, the right to amend or supplement one's PHI, the right to request that a covered entity restrict the use and disclosure of one's PHI for the purposes of treatment, payment, or other health care operations, and the right to an accounting of PHI disclosures (other than for treatment, payment, or health care operations, or pursuant to an authorization).
Minimum Necessary	Covered entities must limit the use, disclosure, or request of PHI, to the extent practicable, to a limited data set or, if needed, to the minimum necessary to accomplish the intended purpose of such use, disclosure, or request. This requirement holds until the Secretary issues guidance on what constitutes minimum necessary. In addition, the Act clarifies that the entity disclosing the PHI (as opposed to the requester) makes the minimum necessary determination. The HIPAA privacy rule's exceptions to the minimum necessary standard continue to apply.	As previously discussed, the privacy rule incorporates a minimum necessary standard. There are a number of circumstances in which the minimum necessary standard does not apply; for example, disclosures to or requests by a health care provider for treatment purposes. The rule also permits the disclosure of a "limited data set" for certain specified purposes (e.g., research), pursuant to a data use agreement with the recipient. A limited data set has most direct identifiers removed and is considered to pose a low privacy risk.

Table 1. (Continued).

Topic	Summary of Provision	Current Requirements and Activities
Sale of Patient Information	The Act prohibits the sale of PHI by a covered entity or business associate without patient authorization except in certain specified circumstances, including: (1) public health activities (as described in 45 CFR 164.512(b)); (2) research (as described in 45 CFR 164.512(i)); (3) treatment of the individual; and (4) providing the individual with a copy of his or her PHI. Within 18 months of enactment, the Secretary must issue he sale of PHI.	Unless expressly permitted or required under the rule, the disclosure of PHI to a third party is prohibited without patient authorization.
Marketing	The Act clarifies that a marketing communication by a covered entity or business associate about a product or service that encourages the recipient to purchase or use the product or service may not be considered a health care operation, unless the communication is for a health care-related product or service, or relates to the treatment of the individual. Further, such a communication about a health-care related product or service may not be considered a health care operation if the covered entity receives payment for the making the communication, unless (1) the communication describes only a drug or biologic that is currently being prescribed for the recipient and the payment is reasonable (as defined by the Secretary), (2) the covered entity obtains authorization from the recipient, or (3) in the event the communication is made by a business associate on behalf of a covered entity, the communication is consistent with the contract.	Generally, a covered entity may not use or disclose health information for its own marketing activities without authorization. However, communications made by a covered entity (or its business associate) to encourage a patient to purchase or use a health care-related product or service are excluded from this definition and, therefore, do not require the patient's authorization, even if the covered entity is paid by a third party to engage in such activities.
Fundraising	Fundraising communications for the benefit of the covered entity must, in a clear and conspicuous manner, provide an opportunity for the recipient to opt out of receiving further communications. Treats a recipient's decision to opt out as equivalent to a revocation of authorization.	A covered entity may use or disclose to a business associate or foundation, for the purposes of fundraising, patient demographic information and dates of health care provided. Fundraising materials must include a description of how the recipient may opt out of further communications. Covered entities must make a reasonable effort to ensure that those who opt out do not receive further communications.

Topic	Summary of Provision	Current Requirements and Activities
Notification of Information Breach: PHR Vendors and Other non-HIPAA Covered Entities	PHR vendors and entities offering products and services through a PHR vendor's website, upon discovery of a breach of security of unsecured PHR health information, must notify the individuals impacted and the Federal Trade Commission (FTC). The previously described requirements for the content and timeliness of notifications apply also to this provision. Unsecured PHR health information means PHR health information that is not protected through the use of a technology or methodology specified in guidance issued by the Secretary. If the Secretary fails to issue guidance, then PHR health information will be considered unsecure if not secured by a technology standard rendering it unusable, unreadable, or indecipherable to unauthorized individuals that was developed or endorsed by a standards development organization accredited by ANSI. The FTC must notify HHS of any breach notices it receives and has enforcement authority regarding such breaches of unsecured PHR health information. Within 180 days, the FTC must issue interim final regulations to implement this section. The provisions in this section will no longer apply if Congress enacts new legislation establishing breach notification requirements for non-HIPAA covered entities.	The privacy and security rules apply to covered entities (i.e., health plans and pro written contracts, to their business associates. As already noted, however, the privacy and security rules do not require covered entities to notify HHS or others of a breach of the privacy, security, or integrity of PHI. However, business associate contracts must include a provision requiring them to report to covered entities if they become aware of any security incident or any use or disclosure of PHI that is not provided for by the contract.
Business Associate Contracts	The Act requires organizations that contract with covered entities for the purpose of exchanging electronic PHI (e.g., Health Information Exchanges, Regional Health Information Organizations (RHIOs), and PHR vendors) to have business associate contracts with those entities.	
Criminal Penalties	The Act amends HIPAA to clarify that criminal penalties for wrongful disclosure of PHI apply to individuals who without authorization obtain or disclose such information maintained by a covered entity, whether they are employees or not.	In July 2005, the Justice Department's Office of Legal Counsel addressed which persons may be prosecuted under HIPAA and concluded that only a covered entity could be criminally liable.
Civil Penalties	The Act amends HIPAA to permit OCR to pursue an investigation and the imposition of civil monetary penalties against any individual for an alleged criminal violation of the HIPAA standards if the Justice Department had not prosecuted the individual. In addition, it amends HIPAA to require a formal investigation of complaints and the imposition of civil monetary penalties for violations due to willful neglect. The Secretary must issue regulations within 18 months to implement those amendments. The Act also requires that any civil monetary penalties collected be transferred to OCR to be used for enforcing the HIPAA privacy and security standards.	As noted above, HIPAA authorized the Secretary to impose civil monetary penalties on any person failing to comply with the privacy and security standards. Civil monetary penalties may not be imposed if: (1) the violation is a criminal offense under HIPAA's criminal penalty provisions; (2) the person did not have actual or constructive knowledge of the violation; or (3) the failure to comply was due to reasonable cause and not to willful neglect, and was corrected within 30 days.

Table 1. (Continued).

Topic	Summary of Provision	Current Requirements and Activities
	Within 18 months of enactment, GAO is required to submit recommendations for giving a percentage of any civil monetary penalties collected to the individuals harmed. Based on those recommendations, the Secretary, within three years of enactment, must establish by regulation a methodology to distribute a percentage of any collected penalties to harmed individuals. The Act further amends HIPAA by replacing the existing civil monetary penalties with four tiers of penalties, the highest of which would impose a fine of $50,000 per violation and up to $1,500,000 for all such violations of an identical requirement or prohibition during a calendar year. It preserves the current requirement that a civil fine not be imposed if the violation was due to reasonable cause and was corrected within 30 days. Finally, state attorneys general are authorized to bring a civil action in federal district court against individuals who violate the HIPAA privacy and security standards. Nothing in the section prevents OCR from continuing to use corrective action without a penalty in cases where the person did not know, and by exercising reasonable diligence would not have known, about the violation.	OCR has not levied a single penalty against a HIPAA-covered entity. Instead, it has focused on working with covered entities to encourage voluntary compliance through corrective action. For certain wr PHI, OCR may refer the case to the Department of Justice for criminal prosecution. HIPAA's criminal penalties include fines of up to $250,000 and up to 10 years in prison for disclosing or obtaining health information with the intent to sell, transfer or use it for commercial advantage, personal gain, or malicious harm.
Compliance Audits	The Secretary is required to perform periodic audits to ensure compliance with the HIPAA privacy and security standards and the requirements of this subtitle.	The Secretary is authorized to conduct compliance reviews to determine whether covered entities are complying with HIPAA standards.
Preemption of State Law	The Act applies the HIPAA preemption provisions to the above privacy requirements and preserves the HIPAA privacy and security standards to the extent that they are consistent with those requirements. The Secretary is required by rulemaking to amend the HIPAA standards as necessary to make them consistent with the Act's privacy and security provisions. The Act does not waive any health privacy privilege otherwise applicable to an individual.	The HIPAA security standards preempt any contrary provision of state law, with certain specified exceptions (e.g., public health reporting). However, the privacy rule does not preempt a contrary provision of state law that is more protective of patient medical privacy.
Effective Date	Except as otherwise specifically provided, the above privacy and security provisions take effect 12 months after enactment.	
Studies, Reports, Guidance	The Secretary is required annually to provide Congress with a compliance report containing information on (1) the number and nature of complaints of alleged violations and how they were resolved, including the imposition of civil fines, (2) the number of covered entities receiving technical assistance in order to achieve compliance, as well as the types of assistance provided, (3) the number of audits performed and a summary of their findings, and (4) the Secretary's plan for the following year for improving compliance with and enforcement of the HIPAA standards and the provisions of this subtitle. In addition, the Secretary is required, within one year and in consultation with FTC, to study the application of health information privacy and security requirements (including breach notification) to non-HIPAA covered entities and report to Congress.	Any person who believes a covered entity is not complying with the privacy rule may file a complaint with HHS. HIPAA does not require the Secretary to issue a compliance report. The privacy and security standards apply to health plans, health care providers, and health care clearinghouses.

Topic	Summary of Provision	Current Requirements and Activities
	The Secretary also is required, within one year of enactment and in consultation with stakeholders, to issue guidance on how best to implement the HIPAA privacy rule's requirements for de-identifying PHI. Finally, the Secretary may, by regulation, revise the definition of psychotherapy notes to include test data that are part of a mental health evaluation. The Act requires GAO, within one year, to report on best practices related to the disclosure of PHI among health care providers for the purpose of treatment. The report must include an examination of practices implemented by states and other entities, such as health information exchanges, and how those practices improve the quality of care, as well as an examination of the use of electronic informed consent for disclosing PHI for treatment, payment, and health care operations. GAO is further required, within five years, to report to Congress and the Secretary on the impact of the Act on health insurance premiums, health care costs, EHR adoption, and improvement in health care quality.	They do not apply directly to other entities that collect and maintain health information, including Health Information Exchanges, RHIOs, and PHR vendors, unless they are acting as providers or plans. The HIPAA standards are intended to protect individually identifiable health information; de-identified information is not subject to the regulations. Under the privacy rule, health information is de-identified if 18 specific identifiers (e.g., name, social security number, address) have been removed, or if a qualified statistician, using accepted principles, determines that the risk if very small that the individual could be identified. Generally, plans and providers may use and disclose health information for the purpose of treatment, payment, and other health care operations without the individual's authorization. Covered entities may, but are not required, to obtain a consent to use or disclose PHI for treatment, payment, or health care operations. Psychotherapy notes (i.e., notes recorded by mental health professionals during counseling) are afforded special protection under the privacy rule. Almost all uses and disclosures of such information require horization.

Source: Table prepared by the Congressional Research Service, based on P.L. 111-5 (Division A, Title XIII), signed by the President on February 17, 2009.

Table 2. HITECH Act: Medicare and Medicaid Payments
American Recovery and Reinvestment Act of 2009 (P.L. 111-5): Division B, Title IV

Topic	Summary of Provision	Current Requirements and Activities
Medicare Incentive Payments and Penalties (Subtitle A)		
Physicians	The Act authorizes incentive payments over a five-year period through Medicare Part B to physicians (as defined in Section 1861(r) of the Social Security Act) who are meaningful users of certified EHR technology. Meaningful use is defined as: (1) demonstrating to the satisfaction of the Secretary the use of certified EHR technology in a meaningful manner (including e-prescribing), including for the purpose of exchanging electronic health information to improve health care quality; and (2) using such certified EHR technology to report clinical quality measures, as selected by the Secretary. The incentive payments equal 75% of the allowed Part B charges during the reporting year. However, the total amount that a physician could receive is capped and decreases over time. Beginning in 2011, eligible physicians will receive up to $15,000 in the first payment year, $12,000 in the second year, $8,000 in the third year, $4,000 in the fourth year, and $2,000 in the fifth, and final, year. Early EHR adopters whose first payment year is 2011 or 2012 will receive up to $18,000 (instead of $15,000) for that year. Eligible physicians first becoming meaningful EHR users after 2013 will receive fewer payments, and those who do not adopt EHRs until after 2014 will receive no bonus. For eligible physicians practicing in health professional shortage areas, the incentive payment amounts are increased by 10%. No incentive payments will be made after 2016. Incentive payments are not available for hospital-based physicians. Eligible physicians who are not meaningful users of certified HIT systems by 2015 will see their Medicare payments reduced by the following amounts: 1% in 2015, 2% in 2016, 3% in 2017 and in each subsequent year. For 2018 and each subsequent year, if the proportion of eligible physicians who are meaningful EHR users is less than 75%, the payment reduction will be further decreased by one percentage point from the applicable amount in the previous year, though the reduction cannot exceed 5%. The Secretary may, on a case-by-case basis, exempt eligible physicians (e.g., rural physicians that lack sufficient Internet access) from the payment reduction if it is determined that being a meaningful EHR user would result in significant hardship. Such exemptions may not be granted for more than five years. Generally, the physician incentive payments are not available to Medicare Advantage (MA) plans. However, the Act provides for the application of the EHR bonus payments and penalties to certain eligible physicians affiliated with MA organizations that function as an HMO.	As previously discussed, CMS is administering a number of programs to promote HIT adoption among health care providers. They include the five-year EHR demonstration, the physician incentive payments for e-prescribing, and the Physician Quality Reporting Initiative (PQRI), under which physicians can earn a bonus for satisfactorily reporting quality measures, including using an EHR.

Topic	Summary of Provision	Current Requirements and Activities
	To avoid duplication of payments, if a physician is both an MA-affiliated provider and eligible for the maximum incentive payment under the fee-for-service (FFS) program, then the payment is to be made only under the FFS program. If the physician is eligible for less than the maximum incentive payment, then the payment is to be made only to the MA organization.	
Hospitals	The Act authorizes incentive payments over a four-year period through Medicare Part A to eligible acute-care hospitals that are meaningful users of certified EHR technology. Meaningful use is defined as: (1) demonstrating to the satisfaction of the Secretary the use of certified EHR technology in a meaningful manner, including for the purpose of exchanging electronic health information to improve health care quality; and (2) using such certified EHR technology to report clinical quality measures, as selected by the Secretary. Beginning in FY2011, eligible hospitals would receive a base amount ($2 million), plus an additional $200 per discharge for the 1,150th through the 23,000th discharge. All payments would be adjusted by the hospital's Medicare share, the value of which takes into account the level of charity care provided (i.e., the more charity care, the higher the Medicare share value). Hospitals would receive the full incentive payment amount in the first fiscal year, 75% in the second fiscal year, 50% in the third fiscal year, and 25% in the fourth, and final, fiscal year. Hospitals that do not become eligible until after FY2015 will receive no payments. Beginning in FY2015: (1) eligible hospitals that failed to report required RHQDAPU quality data would see their market basket (MB) update reduced by one-quarter (i.e., 25%); and (2) eligible hospitals that are not meaningful users of certified EHR systems would see the other three-quarters of their MB update reduced by 33% in FY2015, 67% in FY2016, and 100% in FY2017 and each subsequent fiscal year. The Secretary may, on a case-by-case basis, exempt eligible hospitals (e.g., rural hospitals that lack sufficient Internet access) from the payment reduction if it is determined that being a meaningful EHR user would result in significant hardship. Such exemptions may not be granted for more than five years.	Medicare pays acute care hospitals using a prospectively determined payment for each discharge. These payment rates are increased annually by an update factor that is established in part by the projected increase in the hospital market basket (MB) index. Under the Reporting Hospital Quality Data for Annual Payment Update (RHQDAPU) program, hospitals that do not submit required quality data have the applicable MB percentage reduced by two percentage points. Currently, Medicare's payments to acute care hospitals under the inpatient prospective payment system are not affected by the adoption of EHR.
	Critical access hospitals (CAHs) that are meaningful users of certified EHR technology are eligible for reasonable cost-based reimbursement for the purchase of such technology, based on an enhanced Medicare share that equals the Medicare share calculated for acute-care hospitals for EHR bonuses (see above), including the charity care adjustment, plus an additional 20 percentage points, except the enhanced Medicare share may not exceed 100%. CAHs that are meaningful EHR users may expense these costs in a single payment year and receive prompt interim payments, rather than receiving reimbursement over a multiyear depreciation schedule. Beginning in FY2011, if a CAH is a meaningful EHR user, they are eligible for four consecutive years of payments, except that a CAH cannot get bonuses after FY2015.	Critical access hospitals (CAHs) are limitedservice facilities in rural areas that offer 24-hour emergency care, have no more than 25 acute care inpatient beds, and have a 96-hour average length of stay. Generally, CAHs receive 101% reasonable, cost-based reimbursement for inpatient care provided to Medicare beneficiaries.

Table 2. (Continued).

Topic	Summary of Provision	Current Requirements and Activities
	Beginning in FY2015, CAHs that are not meaningful EHR users would have their Medicare reimbursement rate reduced as follows: for FY2015, 100.66%; for FY2016, 100.33%; and for FY2017 and each subsequent fiscal year, 100%. CAHs are eligible for the same hardship exemption as acute-care hospitals. The EHR payment incentives and penalties also apply to hospitals that are under common corporate governance with a qualifying MA organization and serve enrollees in an MA plan offered by the organization.	
Hold Harmless, Implementation Funding	The Medicare EHR incentive payments are not to be taken into account when calculating Part B premiums or payments rates for MA plans. Monies in the Medicare Improvement Fund may be used to adjust Part B payments to protect against projected shortfalls due to any increase in the conversion factor used to calculate the Part B fee schedule. The Act appropriates $100 million for each of FY2009 through FY2015, and $45 million for FY2016, to implement the above Medicare provisions. The amounts appropriated are to be available until expended.	
HIT Incentive Payment Study	The Secretary is required to conduct a study, and report to Congress by June 30, 2010, on whether EHR payment incentives should be made available to health care providers who are receiving minimal or no payment incentives or other funding under this Act. The study must include an examination of the adoption rates and clinical utility of HER technology by such providers, and the potential costs and benefits of making payment incentives to such providers, among other things.	
Medicaid Funding (Subtitle B)		
EHR Adoption and Operation Payments	The Act authorizes a 100% federal match for payments to certain qualifying Medicaid providers to encourage the adoption and use of certified EHR technology. The 100% federal match applies to 85% of the net average allowable EHR technology costs of a physician, dentist, nurse mid-wife, nurse practitioner, or physician assistant (practicing in a rural clinic of federally qualified heath center led by a physician assistant): (1) who is not hospital-based and has at least a 30% Medicaid patient volume; or (2) who practices predominantly in a federally qualified health center or rural clinic and whose patient volume is at least 30% needy individuals. Pediatricians need only a 20% Medicaid patient volume to be eligible. The 100% federal match also applies to EHR-related payments to children's hospitals, and to other acute-care hospitals with at least a 10% Medicaid patient volume, up to a maximum amount. The state must provide assurances to the Secretary that all allowable costs are paid directly to the provider without any deduction or rebate; that the provider is responsible for payment of the other 15% of HER technology costs; and, that for costs not associated with purchase and initial implementation, the provider demonstrates meaningful use of certified EHR technology.	The federal government pays a share of every state's spending on Medicaid services and program administration. The federal match for administrative expenditures does not vary by state and is generally 50%, but certain functions receive a higher amount. The Medicaid statute authorizes a 90% match for expenditures attributable to the design, development, or installation of mechanized claims processing and information retrieval systems—referred to as Medicaid Management Information Systems (MMISs)—and a 75% match for approved MMIS operations

Topic	Summary of Provision	Current Requirements and Activities
	The Secretary may deem that the establishment of meaningful EHR use for the purpose of Medicare incentive payments is sufficient to qualify as meaningful use under this section. In order to receive Medicaid EHR payments, a provider must waive any right to Medicare EHR incentive payments. For physicians, dentists, nurse mid-wives, nurse practitioners, and qualifying physician assistants who are not hospital-based, the net average allowable costs are to be determined by the Secretary, based on studies submitted by states, but may not exceed: (1) $25,000 in the first year of payment (which may not be later than 2016), intended to cover the purchase and initial implementation of EHR technology; and (2) $10,000 a year thereafter, for a period of up to five years, to cover the costs of EHR operation, maintenance and use. Eligible pediatricians may receive up to two-thirds of those amounts. Allowable costs for children's hospitals and acute-care hospitals are based on the Medicare EHR incentive payment formula, with some modifications. Hospital EHR technology payments may not be made after 2016, unless the provider received a payment for the previous year, and may not be made over a period of more than six years. The Secretary must coordinate the Medicare and Medicaid HIT incentive payments to ensure that physicians and other eligible professionals do not receive duplicate funding. Hospitals, however, may qualify for both. The Act authorizes a 90% federal match for payment to the states to administer the EHR technology payments. The Act further requires that the Secretary periodically submit reports to Congress on the status, progress and oversight of payments to Medicaid providers for EHR technology adoption and operation. The Act appropriates $40 million for each of FY2009 through FY2015 and $20 million for FY2016, to remain available until expended, for administering the EHR technology payments.	. A 50% match is available for nonapproved MMISs. States are required to have an MMIS that meets specified requirements and that the Secretary has found (among other things) is compatible with the claims processing and information retrieval systems used in the administration of the Medicare program.

Source: Table prepared by the Congressional Research Service, based on P.L. 111-5 (Division B, Title IV), signed by the President on F ebruary 17, 2009.

ACKNOWLEDGMENTS

Jim Hahn, Sibyl Tilson, Rich Rimkunas, and Paulette Morgan contributed to this report.

End Notes

[1] Catherine M. DesRoches et al., "Electronic Health Records in Ambulatory Care—A National Survey of Physicians," New England Journal of Medicine, 2008, vol. 359, no. 1, pp. 50-60.

[2] Interoperability refers to the ability of IT systems to share and use electronic information. Sharing clinical data across different HIT applications depends on the use of a standardized format for communicating the information electronically.

[3] The CBO cost estimate for the H.R. 1 conference agreement is at http://www.cbo.gov/ftpdocs/99xx/doc9989/hr1conference.pdf.

[4] U.S. Dept. of Health and Human Services, Office of Inspector General, "Medicare and State Health Programs: Fraud and Abuse; Safe Harbors for Certain Electronic Prescribing and Electronic Health Records Arrangements Under the Anti-Kickback Statute," 71 Federal Register 45110, Aug. 8, 2006. U.S. Dept. of Health and Human Services, Centers for Medicare and Medicaid Services, "Medicare Program: Physicians' Referrals to Health Care Entities With Which They Have Financial Relationships; Exceptions for Certain Electronic Prescribing and Electronic Health Records Arrangements," 71 Federal Register 45140, Aug. 8, 2006.

[5] Unlike an EHR, which is created and controlled by one or more health care providers who populate it with clinical data, a PHR is controlled by the patient. A PHR does not contain the same depth of information as an EHR, and typically includes information from multiple sources, including data on insurance claims. Individuals and other authorized clinical and wellness professionals use the PHR to help guide and make health decisions and manage the patient's care. Many health plans and some employers offer PHRs. Other leading IT companies, including Google and Microsoft, also offer a PHR product.

[6] Those provisions are at the end of Division B, Title IV: (i) Section 4301, Moratoria on Certain Medicare Regulations; and (ii) Section 4302, Long-Term Care Hospital Technical Corrections.

[7] For more details, see CRS Report R40181, *Selected Health Funding in the American Recovery and Reinvestment Act*, coordinated by C. Stephen Redhead.

In: Transforming Healthcare with Health Information… ISBN: 978-1-61324-417-3
Editors: C. M. Denison, E. L. Montevoy

Chapter 3

THE PRIVACY AND SECURITY PROVISIONS FOR HEALTH INFORMATION IN THE AMERICAN RECOVERY AND REINVESTMENT ACT OF 2009*

Gina Stevens and Edward C. Liu

SUMMARY

President Obama signed the American Recovery and Reinvestment Act of 2009 (P.L. 111-5) on February 17, 2009. Title XIII of Division A and Title IV of Division B of that act are referred to as the Health Information Technology for Economic and Clinical Health Act (HITECH Act). The HITECH Act was designed to promote the widespread adoption of health information technology (HIT). HIT involves the exchange of health information in an electronic environment.

The HITECH Act, based on legislation introduced in the 110th Congress, promotes health information technology through codification of the role of the Office of the National Coordinator for Health Information Technology (ONCHIT); adoption of standards for health information technology; creation of grants and loan programs to promote wider HIT use among health care practitioners; and expansion of privacy and security requirements for protected health information. The HITECH Act also includes financial incentives for Medicare and Medicaid health care providers who make meaningful use of electronic health records.

As part of the HITECH Act, sweeping changes to the health information privacy regime were enacted. Most of the provisions in Subtitle D of Title XIII (Privacy) of the HITECH Act are additional requirements supplementing the HIPAA Privacy and Security Rules, but a few provisions deal specifically with electronic health records (EHRs). Subtitle D (Privacy) of Title XIII of the HITECH Act extended application of certain provisions of the HIPAA Privacy and Security Rules to the business associates of covered entities making those business associates subject to civil and criminal liability for violations; established new limits on the use of protected health information for marketing and fundraising purposes; provided new enforcement authority for state attorneys general to bring suit in federal district court to enforce HIPAA violations;

---

* This is an edited, reformatted and augmented version of a Congressional Research Services publication, CRS Report for Congress R40546, from www.crs.gov, dated February 22, 2010.

increased civil and criminal penalties for HIPAA violations; required covered entities and business associates to notify the public or HHS of data breaches (regardless of whether actual harm has occurred); changed certain use and disclosure rules for protected health information; and created additional individual rights.

In this report, we provide an overview of HIPAA, of the HIPAA Privacy and Security Rules, and of the privacy and security provisions for protected health information included in Subtitle D of Title XIII of the HITECH Act.

INTRODUCTION

Over the past two decades, the federal government has undertaken several initiatives to promote health information technology. [1] Health information technology (HIT)[2] involves the exchange of health information in an electronic environment. What began in 1996 with Congress's passage of the Health Insurance Portability and Accountability Act (HIPAA) to facilitate the development of a health information system,[3] was followed in 2004 by President Bush's initiative to make electronic health records (EHRs) available to most Americans within 10 years [4] and the signing of the American Recovery and Reinvestment Act of 2009 (ARRA)[5] by President Obama, which authorized \$22 billion for HIT efforts. Included in ARRA is the Health Information Technology for Economic and Clinical Health Act (HITECH Act) (Title XIII of Division A and Title IV of Division B). The HITECH Act, based on legislation introduced in the 110th Congress,[6] promotes health information technology through codification of the role of the Office of the National Coordinator for Health Information Technology (ONCHIT); adoption of standards for health information technology; creation of grants and loan programs to promote wider HIT use among health care practitioners; and expansion of privacy and security requirements for protected health information. The HITECH Act also includes financial incentives for Medicare and Medicaid health care providers who make meaningful use of electronic health records.

In this report, we provide an overview of HIPAA, of the HIPAA Privacy and Security Rules, and of the privacy and security provisions for protected health information included in Subtitle D of Title XIII of the HITECH Act.[7]

THE HEALTH INSURANCE PORTABILITY AND ACCOUNTABILITY ACT (HIPAA)

Congress enacted the Health Insurance Portability and Accountability Act of 1996 (HIPAA)[8] to "improve portability and continuity of health insurance coverage in the group and individual markets."[9] HIPAA also included tax provisions related to health insurance and administrative simplification provisions[10] requiring "the development of a health information system through the establishment of standards and requirements for the electronic transmission of certain health information."[11] The Department of Health and Human Services (HHS) issued final regulations (such as the HIPAA Privacy and Security Rules) to adopt national standards for transactions and code sets, privacy, security, and employer identifiers.[12] The Office of Civil Rights (OCR) in HHS is responsible for enforcing the Privacy Rule.[13] The

Centers for Medicare and Medicaid Services (CMS) has delegated authority to enforce the non-privacy HIPAA standards, including the Security Rule.[14]

HIPAA applies to covered entities—health plans, health care clearinghouses, and health care providers who transmit financial and administrative transactions electronically.[15] Failure to comply with the regulations may subject the covered entity to civil or criminal penalties.[16] Under HIPAA, the Secretary of HHS is required to impose a civil monetary penalty on any person failing to comply with the national standards and regulations.[17] The maximum civil money penalty (i.e., the fine) for a violation of an administrative simplification provision is $100 per violation and up to $25,000 for all violations of an identical requirement or prohibition during a calendar year.[18] HIPAA also establishes criminal penalties for any person who knowingly and in violation of the Administrative Simplification provisions of HIPAA uses a unique health identifier, or obtains or discloses individually identifiable health information.[19] Enhanced criminal penalties may be imposed if the offense is committed under false pretenses, with intent to sell the information or reap other personal gain. The penalties include (1) a fine of not more than $50,000 and/or imprisonment of not more than one year; (2) if the offense is under false pretenses, a fine of not more than $100,000 and/or imprisonment of not more than five years; and (3) if the offense is with intent to sell, transfer, or use individually identifiable health information for commercial advantage, personal gain, or malicious harm, a fine of not more than $250,000 and/or imprisonment of not more than 10 years.[20] These penalties do not affect other penalties imposed by other federal programs.

The HIPAA preemption rule establishes that any federal regulation resulting from implementation of the act preempts any contrary state law.[21] "Contrary" is defined as situations where (1) a covered entity would find it impossible to comply with both the state and the federal requirements, or (2) when the state law stands as an obstacle to the accomplishment and execution of the full purposes and objectives of Congress.[22]

Congress established three exceptions to this general rule. First, there is an exception for state laws that the Secretary determines are necessary to prevent fraud and abuse, to ensure appropriate state regulation of insurance and health plans, for state reporting on health care delivery, or for other purposes.[23] The second exception provides that state laws will not be superseded if the Secretary determines that the law addresses controlled substances.[24] Both of these exceptions require an affirmative "exception determination" from the Secretary of HHS for the state law not to be preempted.[25] The third exception provides that state laws will not be preempted if they relate to the privacy of individually identifiable health information and are "more stringent" than the federal requirements.[26]

A state law is "more stringent" if it meets one or more of the following criteria: (1) the state law prohibits or further limits the use or disclosure of protected health information, except if the disclosure is required by HHS to determine a covered entity's compliance or is made to the individual who is the subject of the individually identifiable information; (2) the state law provides individuals with a greater right to access or amend their individually identifiable health information; provided, however, HIPAA will not preempt a state law to the extent that it authorizes or prohibits disclosure of protected health information about a minor to a parent, guardian, or person acting in loco parentis of such minor; (3) the state law provides for more information to be disseminated to individuals regarding use and disclosure of their protected health information and rights and remedies; (4) the state law narrows the scope or duration of authorization or consent, increases the privacy protections surrounding authorization and consent, or reduces the coercive effect of the surrounding circumstances;

(5) the state law imposes stricter standards for record keeping or accounting of disclosures; (6) the state law strengthens privacy protections for individuals with respect to any other matter.[27]

In addition to the general rule and exceptions, Congress "carved out" two provisions whereby certain areas of state authority will not be limited or invalidated by HIPAA rules. First, the public health "carve out" saves any law providing for the reporting of disease or injury, child abuse, birth, or death for the conduct of public surveillance, investigation or intervention.[28] The second "carve out" allows states to regulate health plans by requiring the plans to report, or provide access to, information for the purpose of audits, program monitoring and evaluation, or the licensure or certification.[29]

The HIPAA Privacy Rule

The HIPAA Privacy Rule[30] was adopted as the national standard for the protection of individually identifiable health information.[31] Enforcement of the Privacy Rule began on April 14, 2003, except that for small health plans with annual receipts of $5 million or less enforcement began April 2004.

The HIPAA Privacy Rule applies to protected health information (PHI)—that is, individually identifiable health information "created or received by a health care provider, health plan, or health care clearinghouse" that "[r]elates to the ... health or condition of an individual" or to the provision of or payment for health care.[32]

The HIPAA Privacy Rule limits the circumstances under which an individual's protected health information may be used or disclosed by covered entities. A covered entity is permitted to use or disclose protected health information without patient authorization for treatment, payment, or health care operations.[33] For other purposes, a covered entity may only use or disclose PHI with patient authorization subject to certain exceptions.[34] Exceptions permit the use or disclosure of PHI without patient authorization or prior agreement for public health, judicial, law enforcement, and other specialized purposes.[35] In certain situations that would otherwise require authorization, a covered entity may use or disclose PHI without authorization provided that the individual is given the opportunity to object or agree prior to the use or disclosure.[36]

The HIPAA Privacy Rule also provides for accounting of certain disclosures;[37] requires covered entities to make reasonable efforts to disclose only the minimum information necessary;[38] requires most covered entities to provide a notice of their privacy practices;[39] establishes individual rights to review and obtain copies of protected health information;[40] requires covered entities to safeguard protected health information from inappropriate use or disclosure; and gives individuals the right to request changes to inaccurate or incomplete protected health information.[41]

The HIPAA Privacy Rule also requires a covered entity to maintain reasonable and appropriate administrative, technical, and physical safeguards to prevent use or disclosure of protected health information in violation of the Privacy Rule.[42]

The HIPAA Privacy Rule defines a business associate as a person who performs, or assists in the performance of a function or activity involving the use or disclosure of individually identifiable health information on behalf of a covered entity.[43] Business associates also include persons who perform legal, actuarial, accounting, consulting, data aggregation, management, administrative, accreditation, or financial services to or for such covered entity where the provision of the service involves the disclosure of individually identifiable health information from such covered entity or arrangement, or from another business associate of such covered entity or arrangement, to the person.[44] The HIPAA Privacy Rule permits a covered entity to disclose health information to a business associate, or to allow a business associate to create or receive PHI on its behalf, provided the covered entity receives satisfactory written assurances that the business associate will safeguard the information.[45] Covered entities may enter into contractual agreements with their business associates, committing the business associates to provide similar protections for PHI. If a business associate fails to meet its responsibilities under its business associate agreement (BAA), then the covered entity must terminate its contractual relationship with the business associate or report the problem to the Secretary of HHS.[46]

The HIPAA Security Rule

The HIPAA Security Rule, 45 C.F.R. Parts 160 and 164,[47] applies only to protected health information in electronic form (EPHI), and requires a covered entity to maintain administrative, technical, and physical safeguards to ensure the confidentiality, integrity, and availability of all EPHI the covered entity creates, receives, maintains, or transmits. Covered entities must protect against any reasonably anticipated threats or hazards to the security or integrity of such information, and any reasonably anticipated uses or disclosures of such information that are not permitted or required under the Privacy Rule; and ensure compliance by its workforce.[48]

The Security Rule requires covered entities to enter into agreements with business associates who create, receive, maintain or transmit EPHI on their behalf. Under such agreements, the business associate must implement administrative, physical, and technical safeguards that reasonably and appropriately protect the confidentiality, integrity, and availability of the covered entity's electronic protected health information; ensure that its agents and subcontractors to whom it provides the information do the same; and report to the covered entity any security incident of which it becomes aware. The contract must also authorize termination if the covered entity determines that the business associate has violated a material term. A covered entity is not liable for violations by the business associate unless the covered entity knew that the business associate was engaged in a practice or pattern of activity that violated HIPAA, and the covered entity failed to take corrective action.

Subtitle D (Privacy) of the HITECH Act

The Health Information Technology for Economic and Clinical Health Act (HITECH Act) was enacted as Title XIII of Division A (§§ 13001-13424) and Title IV of Division B (§§ 4001-4302) of ARRA and signed into law on February 17, 2009, by President Obama.[49] President Obama views the expanded use of EHRs as integral to both economic stimulation and health care reform:

> To improve the quality of our health care while lowering its cost, we will make the immediate investments necessary to ensure that within five years, all of America's medical records are computerized. This will cut waste, eliminate red tape, and reduce the need to repeat expensive medical tests. But it just won't save billions of dollars and thousands of jobs—it will save lives by reducing the deadly, but preventable, medical errors that pervade our health care system.[50]

As part of this new law, sweeping changes to the health information privacy regime were enacted. Most of the provisions in Subtitle D (Privacy) of Title XIII of the HITECH Act contain additional requirements supplementing the pre-existing HIPAA Privacy and Security Rules, but a few provisions deal specifically with EHRs.[51] Subtitle D (Privacy) of Title XIII of the HITECH Act extended application of certain provisions of the HIPAA Privacy and Security Rules to the business associates of covered entities making those business associates subject to civil and criminal liability for violations; established new limits on the use of protected health information for marketing and fundraising purposes; provided new enforcement authority for state attorneys general to bring suit in federal district court to enforce HIPAA violations; increased civil and criminal penalties for HIPAA violations; required covered entities and business associates to notify the public or HHS of data breaches (regardless of whether actual harm has occurred); changed certain use and disclosure rules for protected health information; and created additional individual rights.

Application of the HIPAA Security Provisions and Penalties to Business Associates

The HITECH Act extends the application of the HIPAA Security Rule's provisions on administrative, physical, and technical safeguards and documentation requirements to business associates of covered entities, making those business associates subject to civil and criminal liability for violations of the HIPAA Security Rule.[52]

Under the HIPAA Security Rule, only covered entities can be held civilly or criminally liable for violations. While business associates are still not technically considered covered entities under HIPAA, they will be subject to the same civil and criminal penalties as a covered entity for Security Rule violations occurring after February 17, 2010.[53] The HITECH Act also requires existing business associate agreements to incorporate the new security requirements added by the HITECH Act.[54] The Secretary is also directed to issue annual guidance on the most effective and appropriate technical safeguards.[55]

Breach Notification

Prior to the enactment of the HITECH Act, neither the HIPAA Privacy nor Security Rule required covered entities or business associates to notify individuals when the security or privacy of their PHI had been compromised. Furthermore, vendors of personal health records (PHRs) were also under no obligation to notify affected individuals or the public after a breach of privacy or security.[56] The HITECH Act imposed such notification requirements on covered entities and business associates. A similar requirement was also imposed on vendors of PHR's.

Definitions

The HITECH Act requires covered entities, business associates, and vendors of PHR's to notify affected individuals in the event of a "breach" of "unsecured protected health information."[57] A "breach" is defined as the "unauthorized acquisition, access, use, or disclosure of protected health information which compromises the security or privacy of such information, except where an unauthorized person to whom such information is disclosed would not reasonably have been able to retain such information."[58] A vendor of PHR is defined as "an entity, other than a covered entity ... that offers or maintains a personal health record."[59] The term "unsecured protected health information" means "protected health information that is not secured through the use of a technology or methodology specified by the Secretary in guidance.[60] The HITECH Act required the HHS Secretary to issue initial guidance by April 17, 2009, and annually thereafter specifying the technologies and methodologies that render protected health information unusable, unreadable, or indecipherable to unauthorized individuals.[61] The HITECH Act also provides a default definition if such guidance is not issued. Under the default definition, PHI is unsecured if

> it is not secured by a technology standard that renders protected health information unusable, unreadable, or indecipherable to unauthorized individuals and that is developed or endorsed by a standards developing organization that is accredited by the American National Standards Institute.

On April 17, 2009, guidance on the meaning of "unsecured protected health information " was issued by HHS.[62] It identified two methods for rendering PHI unusable, unreadable, or indecipherable to unauthorized individuals: encryption and destruction (paper and electronic form). Pursuant to this guidance, "if PHI is rendered unusable, unreadable, or indecipherable to unauthorized individuals by one or more of the methods identified in this guidance, then such information is not "unsecured" PHI. Thus, because the breach notification requirements apply only to breaches of unsecured PHI, this guidance provides the means by which covered entities and their business associates are to determine whether a breach has occurred [and the extent] to which the notification obligations under the Act and its implementing regulations apply."[63]

Notice of Unauthorized Disclosure of Protected Health Information

Section 13402 of the HITECH Act requires a covered entity to notify affected individuals when it discovers that their unsecured PHI has been, or is reasonably believed to have been, breached.[64] This requirement applies to covered entities that access, maintain, retain, modify, record, store, destroy, or otherwise hold, use, or disclose unsecured protected health information. The scope of notification is dependant upon the number of individuals whose unsecured PHI was compromised. Generally, only written notice need be provided if less than 500 individuals are involved.[65] For larger breaches, notice through prominent media outlets may be required. In all cases, the Secretary of HHS must be notified, although breaches involving less than 500 people may be reported on an annual basis. The Secretary of HHS is directed to display on the department's website a list of covered entities with breaches involving more than 500 individuals.[66]

Generally, notice must be given without unreasonable delay, but no later than 60 days after the breach is discovered. If a delay is not reasonable, a covered entity may still have violated this provision even if notice was given within 60 days. In an enforcement action of this provision, the covered entity has the burden of proving that any delay was reasonable. Delayed notification is permitted for law enforcement purposes if a law enforcement official determines that notice would impede a criminal investigation or cause damage to national security.

To the extent possible, notification of a breach must include a description of what occurred, a description of the types of information involved in the breach, steps individuals should take in response to the breach, a description of what the covered entity is doing to investigate, mitigate, and protect against further harm, and contact information to obtain additional information.

The Secretary is required to annually submit a report to Congress containing information on the number and nature of breaches for which notice was provided, and actions taken in response to such breaches.[67] HHS issued an interim final rule on August 24, 2009, to implement the breach notification requirement.[68]

Notice of Unauthorized Disclosure of Personal Health Records

Section 13407 of the HITECH Act includes a temporary breach notification requirement for PHR vendors (such as Google Health or Microsoft Vault), service providers to PHR vendors, and PHR servicers that are not covered entities or business associates that sunsets "if Congress enacts new legislation."[69] Under the temporary requirement, these entities are required to notify citizens and residents of the United States whose unsecured "PHR identifiable health information" has been, or is believed to have been, breached. PHR vendors, service providers to PHR vendors, and PHR servicers are also required to notify the federal government, although in this case the governing agency is the Federal Trade Commission (FTC) and not HHS.[70]

The HITECH Act defines several terms specific to the PHR breach notification requirement. A "breach of security" is defined as the unauthorized acquisition of an individual's PHR identifiable health information.[71] PHR identifiable health information is defined as individually identifiable health information, and includes information provided by or on behalf on the individual, and information that can reasonably be used to identify the individual.[72]

The requirements regarding the scope, timing, and content of these notifications are identical to the requirements applicable to breaches of PHI under § 13402 of the HITECH Act. Violations of these requirements shall be considered unfair and deceptive trade practices in violation of the Federal Trade Commission Act.[73]

The HITECH Act also directed the FTC to issue regulations implementing these requirements by August 18, 2009. Final rules issued by the FTC would apply to breaches that are discovered after September 24, 2009, by vendors of PHRs, service providers to PHR vendors, and PHR servicers.[74] The rule also contains provisions discussing the breach notification requirement, the timeliness of notification, methods of notification, content of notifications, and enforcement of these requirements.

Health Information Privacy Education

Section 13403 of the HITECH Act directs the Secretary of HHS to designate a privacy advisor for each regional office of HHS, who will offer guidance and education to covered entities, business associates, and individuals on their rights and obligations regarding PHI.[75] The OCR is also directed to develop within a year of enactment a multilingual national education initiative to enhance public transparency and educate the public about the potential uses of their protected health information.[76]

Application of HIPAA Privacy Provisions and Penalties to Business Associates

Section 13404 of the HITECH Act provides that covered entities' business associates that obtain or create PHI pursuant to a business associate agreement (BAA) may only use or disclose that PHI in compliance with the terms of that BAA.[77] The HITECH Act also requires existing business associate agreements to incorporate the new privacy provisions added by the HITECH Act.[78]

In some cases, an entity or individual may be held liable for the HIPAA violations of another. Covered entities have been liable for violations of the Privacy Rule that were committed by their business associates, but only if the covered entity had knowledge of "a pattern of activity or practice" of the business associate that violates the Privacy Rule.[79] Under the HITECH Act, this vicarious liability remains, and business associates are made reciprocally liable for violations of the Privacy Rule committed by covered entities with which they contract, if the business associates are aware of a pattern and practice of unlawful conduct by the covered entity.[80]

While business associates are still not technically considered covered entities under HIPAA, they will be subject to the same civil and criminal penalties as any person for improper uses or disclosures of PHI that occur after February 17, 2010.[81]

Individual Rights Regarding Protected Health Information

The HITECH Act includes several provisions that provide individuals with more direct control and oversight over their PHI. Individuals would be able to restrict certain disclosures of PHI and obtain an accounting of all PHI disclosures made from an EHR within the last three years. Additionally, the HITECH Act would explicitly require the content of disclosures to be restricted to avoid disclosure of information that is not necessary for the purpose of the disclosure.

Restrictions on Disclosures

Section 13405(a) of the HITECH Act gives individuals the right to restrict disclosures of PHI that pertain solely to items or services for which the provider has been paid out of pocket in full, if the disclosures were to be made to a health plan for payment or health care operations and is not otherwise required by law.

Minimum Necessary

The HIPAA Privacy Rule requires covered entities to "make reasonable efforts to limit protected health information to the minimum information necessary to accomplish the intended purpose of the use, disclosure, or request."[82]

The HIPAA Privacy Rule also permits the use or disclosure of a limited data set for research, public health, or health care operations.[83] A limited data set is defined as PHI that excludes 16 direct identifiers of individuals including names, addresses, social security numbers, email addresses, web URL addresses, and biometric identifiers.[84]

Section 13405(b) of the HITECH Act requires covered entities and business associates to restrict the uses, disclosures, or requests of PHI to a limited data set, to the extent practicable. If this is not practicable, the minimum necessary information may be used or disclosed to accomplish the intended use, disclosure, or request.[85] The Secretary is directed to issue guidance on what information may be considered minimally necessary.[86] The requirement to use only the limited data set, to the extent practicable, sunsets at such time as the Secretary issues guidance on what constitutes minimum necessary.[87] The HITECH Act clarifies that the entity making a disclosure, and not the recipient of the information, would be the one to determine what information was minimally necessary.[88]

Requesting an Accounting

The HITECH Act also gives individuals expanded rights to an accounting of PHI disclosures made by a covered entity that uses electronic health records. Under current law, an individual has a right to such an accounting for the previous six years, but the covered entity is not required to include disclosures made for treatment, payment, or health care operations purposes.[89] Section 13405(c) requires an accounting of these disclosures provided that the covered entity uses electronic health records. Disclosures for treatment, payment, or health care operations need only be tabulated for the previous three years.

The effective date of this provision depends upon whether a covered entity has already adopted electronic health records. For covered entities that adopted EHRs before February 17, 2009, this provision will apply to disclosures made after January 1, 2014. For covered entities that have not already adopted EHRs, it will apply to disclosures made from an EHR after January 1, 2011, or the actual date when an EHR system is implemented, whichever is later. The delayed effective date for covered entities that already use EHRs may be to accommodate entities that had implemented EHRs before they had notice that this expanded accounting requirement would be imposed. The Secretary of HHS may delay applicability of this provision in either case by up to three years.[90]

Sales of Protected Health Information

Under the Privacy Rule, if a covered entity is being directly or indirectly paid to use or disclose PHI for a marketing purpose, it must notify the individual of that payment in addition to getting prior authorization.[91]

Section 13405(d) of the HITECH Act further requires covered entities and business associates to obtain prior authorization from an individual before using or disclosing PHI in exchange for direct or indirect remuneration.[92] Unlike the requirement in the Privacy Rule described above, the HITECH Act requirement is not restricted to marketing communications. However, prior authorization before receiving remuneration is not required when transferring PHI for research activities,[93] when transferring PHI for the treatment of the individual,[94] when transferring PHI to the individual pursuant to his request,[95] or when transferring PHI for use in public health activities.[96]

The HITECH Act directs the Secretary to consider whether limiting such payments to reflect the costs of preparation and transmittal would have an adverse impact on public health activities.[97] If no adverse impact is anticipated, the Secretary may issue regulations imposing limits on payments in the context of public health activities.[98]

Many business associates may transfer PHI for legitimate purposes, at the request of covered entities pursuant to a BAA. In these cases, business associates may also be paid by covered entities for these services. While the business associate could be considered to be receiving indirect remuneration in exchange for transferring PHI in this case, this situation is explicitly exempted from the prior authorization requirement under the HITECH Act.[99] The receipt of any remuneration in exchange for PHI in the context of a merger involving a covered entity also does not require prior authorization.[100]

The Secretary may also create, through regulations, other exceptions that are consistent with the statutory exceptions.[101] This prior authorization requirement will apply to transfers that occur six months after the Secretary promulgates regulations implementing this subsection.[102]

Access to EHRs

Section 13405(e) of the HITECH Act requires covered entities that maintain EHRs to provide individuals an electronic copy of their health records. The individual may also direct the covered entity to transmit the EHR to another entity or person designated by the individual. A covered entity may pass any labor costs associated with either transfer along to the individual.103

Restrictions on Commercial Uses of Protected Health Information

Several provisions of the HITECH Act also restrict certain specific uses and disclosures of PHI for marketing and fundraising purposes. Each of these provisions is discussed below.

Marketing

Section 13406(a) of the HITECH Act made changes to the ways in which PHI may be used for marketing communications. These changes will apply to communications made after February 17, 2010.[104] The Privacy Rule defines marketing as any communication "about a product or service that encourages recipients of the communication to purchase or use the product or service."[105] However, this definition excludes communications

> (i) To describe a health-related product or service (or payment for such product or service) that is provided by, or included in a plan of benefits of, the covered entity making the communication, including communications about: the entities participating in a health care provider network or health plan network; replacement of, or enhancements to, a health plan; and health-related products or services available only to a health plan enrollee that add value to, but are not part of, a plan of benefits.
>
> (ii) For treatment of the individual; or

(iii) For case management or care coordination for the individual, or to direct or recommend alternative treatments, therapies, health care providers, or settings of care to the individual.[106]

Any use or disclosure of PHI for a marketing communication must have the prior authorization of the individual to which the PHI pertains, "notwithstanding any provision of" the Privacy Rule.[107]

Generally, the Privacy Rule permits covered entities to use and disclose PHI for the purpose of treatment, payment, and other health care operations without the individual's authorization and with few restrictions. Health care operations are broadly defined to include quality assessment and improvement activities, case management and care coordination, evaluation of health care professionals, underwriting, legal services, business planning, customer services, grievance resolution, and fundraising. The HITECH Act does not make any changes to the definition of marketing or the prior authorization requirement. However, it does provide that a communication that meets the definition of marketing may not be considered a health care operation.[108] Section 13406(a) of the HITECH Act clarifies that all uses or disclosures of PHI for marketing communications require prior authorization.

As described above, a communication is not considered marketing under the Privacy Rule if it meets one of three exceptions. However, the HITECH Act further provides that, if a communication which qualifies for one of these exceptions was made in exchange for direct or indirect payment, that communication shall not be considered a health care operation.[109] Therefore, these communications, which are not technically considered marketing under the Privacy Rule, may nevertheless require prior authorization unless they are made for treatment, payment, or one of the other exceptions identified in the Privacy Rule.

An exception to this restriction on communications made for payment permits communications that describe drugs or biologics that are currently being prescribed to the recipient of the communication.[110] This protection only applies if the payment is reasonable in amount.[111] These communications may still be considered a health care operation, even when made in exchange for payment. For example, a doctor could receive reasonable payments from a drug manufacturer to provide patients with refill reminders without obtaining prior authorization from the patient. The Secretary is empowered to define reasonable payment through regulation.[112]

Business associates may also make communications on behalf of covered entities pursuant to the terms of the business associate agreement governing that relationship.[113] Because such agreements are required to incorporate the new requirements of the HITECH Act, business associates are subject to the same restrictions regarding marketing communications.

Fundraising

The HIPAA Privacy Rule generally permits covered entities to use or disclose protected health information (PHI) for treatment, payment, or health care operations without prior authorization.[114] The definition of "health care operations" includes "fundraising for the benefit of the covered entity."[115] Therefore, prior authorization may not be required before using PHI for fundraising activities. However, a covered entity must give notice to individuals indicating that the covered entity may use PHI for fundraising purposes.[116] The covered entity may only use demographic information about the individual, or the dates on which health care was provided to the individual.[117] Any fundraising materials must also provide the individual with instructions on how to "opt out" of future fundraising communications.[118]

Under § 13406(b) of the HITECH Act, changes to the fundraising provisions of the HIPAA Privacy Rule took effect on February 17, 2010. That section provides,

> The Secretary shall by rule provide that any written fundraising communication that is a healthcare operation as defined under section 164.501 of title 45, Code of Federal Regulations, shall, in a clear and conspicuous manner, provide an opportunity for the recipient of the communications to elect not to receive any further such communication. When an individual elects not to receive any further such communication, such election shall be treated as a revocation of authorization under section 164.508 of title 45, Code of Federal Regulations.

This section reiterates the "opt out" requirement that is currently in place and additionally requires the "opt out" language be "clear and conspicuous." Furthermore, the conference report language discussing this section indicates that it was included to provide certain protections to individuals who opt out, including "the right not to be denied treatment as a result of making that choice."[119] The House version of the HITECH Act included a provision that would have prohibited fundraising communications without prior written authorization, but that language does not appear to have been included in the final legislation.[120]

Business Associate Contracts Required for Certain Entities

Because the current landscape of electronic health information exchange poses new issues and involves additional organizations (such as health information exchange organizations or regional health information organizations) that were not contemplated at the time the HIPAA Privacy and Security Rules were drafted, Subtitle D (Privacy) of the HITECH Act was written in part to address these developments. Section 13408 of the HITECH Act provides that for each organization that provides data transmission of PHI and that needs routine access to PHI, the organization is required to enter into a business associate agreement with a covered entity and will be considered a business associate of the covered entity for purposes of the HIPAA Privacy and Security Rules.[121] Examples of such organizations include Health Information Exchange Organizations, Regional Health Information Organizations, E-prescribing Gateways, and vendors that contract with a covered entity to provide PHRs to patients.[122]

Application of Criminal Penalties

Section 13409 of the HITECH Act amends HIPAA to clarify that any person (including employees of covered entities) may be subject to criminal penalties for obtaining or disclosing protected health information that is maintained by a covered entity.[123] This criminal liability applies to persons that would not be considered covered entities for purposes of HIPAA.

Enforcement

The HITECH Act includes several provisions to provide greater enforcement of the HIPAA Privacy and Security Rules. These provisions increase civil and criminal penalties and give authority to state attorneys general to bring enforcement suits for violations of the Privacy or Security Rules. The enforcement provisions are a fundamental change to the HIPAA enforcement scheme. This is likely in response to what was perceived by some to be lax enforcement of the civil and criminal liability provisions by HHS and DOJ.[124] Each of these provisions is discussed in more detail below.

Enforcement by the Office of Civil Rights

Section 13410(a) of the HITECH Act will give OCR expanded authority to bring suit seeking civil monetary penalties for violations of the HIPAA Privacy or Security Rules and the new requirements of the HITECH Act. This authority will apply to penalties applied on or after February 27, 2011.[125] Prior to the enactment of the HITECH Act, OCR was not authorized to seek civil monetary penalties against an individual if the offense is also punishable as a criminal violation of HIPAA, which would be prosecutable by the Department of Justice.[126] Under the HITECH Act, this limitation will be reduced to cases in which a criminal penalty was actually imposed for the violation.[127] Therefore, OCR will have the authority to seek civil monetary penalties in cases in which criminal prosecution was previously available, but was not pursued.

Section 13410(a) of the HITECH Act also requires the Secretary to impose a civil monetary penalty in cases where a violation of the HIPAA Privacy or Security Rules, or the new requirements of the HITECH Act, were due to willful neglect.[128]

Section 13410(c) provides that the proceeds of any civil monetary penalties or settlements will be transferred to the OCR to fund enforcement of the HIPAA Privacy and Security Rules and the HITECH Act. The Comptroller General is directed to recommend methodologies by which a percentage of the collected funds can be given to harmed individuals. The Secretary of HHS is directed to establish such a methodology by regulation within three years of the recommendation by the Comptroller General.

Increased Civil Monetary Penalties

Section 13410(d) of the HITECH Act creates a new tiered system of civil monetary penalties, based upon how knowing or willful a violation is. Each tier establishes a minimum fine that may be imposed, but also gives the Secretary the discretion to impose a maximum fine of $50,000 per violation, not to exceed $1.5 million in the aggregate for an identical type of violation in one calendar year.[129] Because this maximum fine is available in all cases, regardless of a person's intent, the HITECH Act greatly increases the potential civil monetary liability of covered entities and business associates.

The lowest tier applies to persons that had no knowledge that they committed a violation, and also would not have known had they exercised reasonable diligence. The minimum fine for these persons is $100 per violation, not to exceed $25,000 in the aggregate per year.[130]

The maximum fine is $50,000 per violation, or $1.5 million in the aggregate per year. If actions are taken to correct the violation within 30 days after the violation is discovered, no penalty can be assessed.[131]

The middle tier applies to violations that were due to reasonable cause, and not willful neglect. The minimum fine for these violations is $1,000 per violation, not to exceed $100,000 in the aggregate per year.[132] The maximum fine is $50,000 per violation, or $1.5 million in the aggregate per year. If actions are taken to correct the violation within 30 days after the violation is discovered, no penalty can be assessed. [133]

The highest civil penalties are reserved for violations that are due to willful neglect. The minimum fine for these violations is $10,000 per violation, not to exceed $250,000 per year, if the violation is corrected within 30 days of date the violation was discovered or would have been discovered through reasonable diligence.[134] The maximum fine is $50,000 per violation, or $1.5 million in the aggregate per year. If no corrective action is taken, the minimum fine is identical to the maximum fine: $50,000 per violation, not to exceed $1.5 million in the aggregate per year.[135]

State Attorney General Enforcement

Section 13410(e)(1) of the HITECH Act amends § 1176 of the Social Security Act to create a new subsection (d). The new § 1176(d)(1) states that

> in any case in which the attorney general of a State has reason to believe that an interest of one or more of the residents of that State has been or is threatened or adversely affected by any person who violates a provision of [the HIPAA Privacy or Security rules], the attorney general of the State, as parens patriae, may bring a civil action on behalf of such residents of the State in a district court of the United States of appropriate jurisdiction—(A) to enjoin further such violation by the defendant; or (B) to obtain [statutory] damages on behalf of such residents of the State.

Prior to the enactment of this provision, only the Secretary of HHS was permitted to pursue civil enforcement for violations of the Privacy or Security Rules. The statute did not provide a private cause of action for individuals harmed by HIPAA privacy and security violations.[136] The enforcement authority given to state attorneys general under this provision only applies to violations which occur after the date of the HITECH Act's enactment[137] and is subject to the same six-year statute of limitations as civil monetary penalties sought by the Secretary of HHS for HIPAA violations.[138] The state attorney general bringing such an action must also give notice to the Secretary of HHS, who may intervene.[139] An action by a state attorney general may not be brought while a federal action is pending.[140]

Section 1176(d) provides statutory damages of $100 per violation, not to exceed $25,000 for each category of HIPAA privacy or security provisions violated. For example, if a covered entity sent fundraising solicitations to 300 individuals that had previously opted out of such communications, the maximum statutory fine that could be sought by a state attorney general would be $25,000 not $30,000. Actions brought by state attorneys general may also seek reasonable attorney fees.[141]

One question that may be raised by § 1176(d) is whether this provision also authorizes state attorneys general to bring suit in state courts. The Supreme Court has held that state courts enjoy "a presumption of concurrent jurisdiction" to enforce federal law, and that this presumption may only be rebutted "by an explicit statutory directive, by unmistakable implication from legislative history, or by a clear incompatibility between state-court jurisdiction and federal interests."[142]

In analyzing whether Congress has sought to limit the concurrent jurisdiction of state courts, it is common to first look to the text of the statute to see if Congress has expressly spoken on the matter. The text of § 1176(d) states that "the attorney general of [a] State, as parens patriae, *may* bring a civil action on behalf of such residents of the State in a district court of the United States of appropriate jurisdiction."[143] Although a federal district court of appropriate jurisdiction is the only forum identified in the statute, the Supreme Court has previously held that a permissive grant of jurisdiction to federal courts is not a sufficiently explicit statement to divest the state courts of concurrent jurisdiction. For example, in *Tafflin v. Levitt*, the Court held that a federal statute providing that "'any person injured in his business or property by reason of a violation of [the Racketeer Influenced and Corrupt Organizations Act (RICO)] *may* sue therefor in any appropriate United States district court'" was plainly permissive and not mandatory, "for 'the statute does not state nor even suggest that such jurisdiction shall be exclusive.'"[144]

An examination of the legislative history of § 1176(d) does not provide any indication that Congress intended to restrict or permit the jurisdiction of state courts over these claims. The conference report for P.L. 111-5 states simply that this provision would "authorize State Attorneys General to bring a civil action in Federal district court against individuals who violate the HIPAA privacy and security standards."[145] Similarly, neither the House nor Senate reports on companion bills, each with similar provisions regarding the enforcement authority of state attorneys general, provide any additional illumination of Congress's intent on this point.[146] A search of the Congressional Record did not find any discussion or debate of this provision by members of either the House or Senate that provided any insight on the exclusivity of federal jurisdiction.[147]

Even with no express language in either the statutory text or the legislative history of the provision supporting exclusive federal jurisdiction, a court might still be convinced that allowing states to retain concurrent jurisdiction would be incompatible with the purpose behind a federal statute. In *Gulf Offshore Company v. Mobil Oil Corporation*, the Supreme Court identified three factors which argue for exclusive federal jurisdiction: "the desirability of uniform interpretation, the expertise of federal judges in federal law, and the assumed greater hospitality of federal courts to peculiarly federal claims."[148]

The latter two factors, the expertise of federal judges and greater hospitality of federal courts to peculiarly federal claims, do not seem to be implicated in the case of HIPAA. Many states have enacted laws which provide similar protections for private medical information, and these claims are frequently resolved by the various state court systems. There are no obvious reasons to believe that federal courts would have more expertise in these issues or would be more hospitable to these claims than state courts.

The circumstances of HIPAA more strongly implicate the first factor, namely the desirability of promoting a uniform interpretation of federal law. A uniform interpretation of HIPAA is more likely, but still far from certain, under twelve federal circuits than with the addition of fifty distinct state court systems. On the other hand, uniformity was not found to be a sufficient justification for implying exclusive federal jurisdiction with respect to a number of other federal statutory schemes such as, RICO,[149] Title VII of the Civil Rights Act 1964,[150] and the Labor Management Relations Act of 1947.[151] It is not clear why HIPAA would require more uniformity than any of these other statutes for which concurrent state jurisdiction was upheld.

However, even if an action by state attorneys general under § 13410(e) is initially brought in a state court, it may still end up in federal court through the process of removal. Federal law gives defendants in state court the option of transferring their case to a federal district court, if it would have been proper to bring the action in federal court in the first place.[152] Because the federal district courts have jurisdiction under § 13410(e) to hear actions by state attorneys general enforcing HIPAA violations, defendants in state court would appear have the option of removing these cases to federal court.

On January 12, 2010, the Attorney General of Connecticut brought the first suit under this provision. The suit alleges violations of various provisions of the HIPAA Security and Privacy Rules in connection with the loss of a portable computer drive containing PHI for over 400,000 persons.[153]

Audits

Section 13411 of the HITECH Act directs the Secretary to provide for periodic audits to ensure that covered entities and business associates are in compliance with the HIPAA Privacy and Security Rules, and the HITECH Act.[154]

Relationship to Other Laws

With respect to state laws, the HITECH Act preempts contrary provisions of state law in the same manner as the federal regulations promulgated under HIPAA.[155] The Secretary of HHS is directed to use the regulatory process to bring any inconsistent provisions into alignment with the HITECH Act.[156] Any other provisions that are not inconsistent with the HITECH Act will continue to remain in effect.[157]

Studies, Reports, and Guidance

Section 13424 of the HITECH Act directs the Secretary to annually submit a report to Congress concerning the complaints of alleged violations of the HIPAA Privacy and Security Rules or the HITECH Act.[158] This report must include the number of complaints, the number resolved informally, the number of civil monetary penalties assessed, the number of compliance reviews, the number of subpoenas issued, the Secretary's plan for improving compliance, and the number of audits performed.[159] The Secretary is also directed to conduct a study on privacy and security requirements of entities that are not subject to HIPAA;[160] to issue guidance on how to implement de-identification requirements of the HIPAA Privacy Rule by February 17, 2010;[161] and to conduct a study on the definition of "psychotherapy notes" under the HIPAA Privacy Rule.[162]

Section 13424 of the HITECH Act also directs the Government Accountability Office to submit a report to Congress on the best practices related to the disclosure of PHI for treatment purposes,[163] and a report on the effect of the HITECH Act on health insurance premiums, overall health care costs, adoption of EHRs, and the reduction of medical errors.[164]

End Notes

[1] In 2008, the HHS Office of the National Coordinator (ONC) for Health Information Technology released a "Nationwide Privacy and Security Framework For Electronic Exchange of Individually Identifiable Health Information." *See* http://www.hhs.gov/healthit/documents/NationwidePS_Framework.pdf (Dec. 15, 2008). In addition, the HHS Office for Civil Rights (OCR) recently published two new HIPAA Privacy Rule guidance documents: the HIPAA Privacy Rule's Right of Access and Health Information Technology (http://www.hhs.gov/ocr/privacy/hipaa/ understanding/special/healthit/eaccess.pdf) and Personal Health Records and the HIPAA Privacy Rule.

[2] "The term 'health information technology' means hardware, software, integrated technologies or related licenses, intellectual property, upgrades, or packaged solutions sold as services that are designed for or support the use by health are entities or patients for the electronic creation, maintenance, access, or exchange of health information." P.L. 111-5, § 13101.

[3] P.L. 104-191.

[4] Executive Order 13335: *Incentives for the Use of Health Information Technology and Establishing the Position of the National Health Information Technology Coordinator, (2004).* Health and Human Services and the National Coordinator for Health IT, *The Decade of Health Information Technology: Delivering Consumer-centric and Information-rich Health Care, Framework for Strategic Action* (July 21, 2004), available at http://www.hhs.gov/healthit/documents/hitframework.pdf.

[5] P.L. 111-5.

[6] S. 1693, The Wired for Health Care Quality Act; H.R. 6357, the PRO(TECH)T Act of 2008; and H.R. 6898, the Health-e Information Technology Act of 2008.

[7] For information on the HITECH Act in its entirety, see CRS Report R40161, *The Health Information Technology for Economic and Clinical Health (HITECH) Act*, by C. Stephen Redhead.

[8] P.L. 104-191, 110 Stat. 1936 (1996), codified in part at 42 U.S.C. §§ 1320d *et seq.*

[9] H.Rept. 104-496, at 1, 66-67, reprinted in 1996 U.S.C.C.A.N. 1865, 1865-66.

[10] 42 U.S.C. §§ 1320d—1320d-8.

[11] 110 Stat. 2021.

[12] 42 U.S.C. §§ 1320d-2(a)-(d). *See* CRS Report R40161, *The Health Information Technology for Economic and Clinical Health (HITECH) Act*, by C. Stephen Redhead, at 2-5.

[13] 65 Fed. Reg. 82381.

[14] 68 Fed. Reg. 60694.

[15] 42 U.S.C. § 1320d-4(b) Requires compliance with the regulations within a certain time period by "each person to whom the standard or implementation specification [adopted or established under Sections 1320d-1 and 1320d-2] applies."

[16] CRS Report RL33989, *Enforcement of the HIPAA Privacy and Security Rules*, by Gina Stevens.

[17] 42 U.S.C. § 1320d-5(a).

[18] 42 U.S.C. § 1320d-5(a)(1).

[19] 42 U.S.C. § 1320d-6.

[20] 42 U.S.C. § 1320d-6(b).

[21] 42 U.S.C. § 1320d-7(a)(1).

[22] 45 C.F.R. 160.202.

[23] 42 U.S.C. § 1320d-7(a)(2)(A)(i).

[24] 42 U.S.C. § 1320d-7(a)(2)(A)(ii).

[25] See 45 C.F.R. 160.203(a), 160.204.

[26] 42 U.S.C. § 1320d-7(a)(2)(B) in conjunction with 42 U.S.C. 1320d-2 note (Section 264(c)(2) of P.L. 104-191).

[27] See 45 C.F.R. 160.202.

[28] 42 U.S.C. 1320d-7(b).

[29] 42 U.S.C. 1320d-7(c).

[30] 45 C.F.R. Parts 160 and 164.

[31] The Privacy Rule went into effect on April 14, 2001. On August 14, 2002, HHS published a modified Privacy Rule. 67 Fed. Reg. 53181 available at http://www.hhs.gov/ocr/hipaa/finalreg.html.
[32] 45 C.F.R. § 160.103.
[33] 45 C.F.R. § 164.506.
[34] 45 C.F.R. § 164.508.
[35] 45 C.F.R. § 164.512(a)-(l).
[36] 45 C.F.R. § 164.510.
[37] 45 C.F.R. § 164.528.
[38] 45 C.F.R. § 164.502(b).
[39] 45 C.F.R. § 164.520.
[40] 45 C.F.R. § 164.524.
[41] 45 C.F.R. § 164.526.
[42] 45 C.F.R. § 164.530(c).
[43] Examples of such activities include claims processing or administration, data analysis, processing or administration, utilization review, quality assurance, billing, benefit management, practice management, and repricing.
[44] 45 C.F.R. § 160.103.
[45] 45 C.F.R. § 164.502(e)(1).
[46] 45 C.F.R. § 164.504(e)(1)(ii).
[47] HIPAA Security Standards for the Protection of Electronic Personal Health Information, 45 C.F.R. Part 164.302 *et seq.*
[48] 45 C.F.R. § 164.306(a).
[49] P.L. 111-5.
[50] President-Elect Urges Electronic Medical Records in 5 Years, George Mason University, Fairfax, VA (Jan. 8, 2009), http://abcnews.go.com/Health/President44/Story?id=6606536&page=1.
[51] An electronic health record is defined as "an electronic record of health-related information on an individual that is created, gathered, managed, and consulted by authorized health care clinicians and staff." P.L. 111-5, § 13400(5).
[52] P.L. 111-5, § 13401. The HITECH Act adopts the same definition of business associates as the HIPAA Privacy and Security Rules. 45 C.F.R. § 160.103.
[53] P.L. 111-5, §§ 13401(b), 13404(c).
[54] P.L. 111-5, § 13404(a).
[55] P.L. 111-5, § 13401(c).
[56] A PHR is defined as an electronic record of identifiable health information on an individual that can be drawn from multiple sources and that is managed, shared, and controlled by or primarily for the individual." P.L. 111-5, § 13400(11). A vendor of PHR is defined as "an entity, other than a covered entity ... that offers or maintains a personal health record." P.L. 111-5, § 13400(18).
[57] P.L. 111-5, §§ 13402, 13407.
[58] P.L. 111-5,§ 13400(1). Not included in the definition of breach are any unintentional acquisition, use, or access of PHI by an employee or other authorized individual of a covered entity or a business associate done in good faith and within the scope of employment or the relationship where such information is not breached any further; or inadvertent disclosures by authorized persons of PHI within the same facility; and information received as a result of such disclosure is not further disclosed without authorization.
[59] P.L. 111-5, § 13400(18).
[60] P.L. 111-5, § 13402(h).
[61] P.L. 111-5, § 13402(h).
[62] HHS, *Guidance Specifying the Technologies and Methodologies That Render Protected Health Information Unusable, Unreadable, or Indecipherable to Unauthorized Individuals for Purposes of the Breach Notification Requirements under Section 13402 of Title XIII (Health Information Technology for Economic and Clinical Health Act) of the American Recovery and Reinvestment Act of 2009*, at 2, available at http://www.hhs.gov/ocr/privacy/hipaa/understanding/coveredentities/hitechrfi.pdf.
[63] *Id.* at 15-16.
[64] P.L. 111-5, § 13402(a).
[65] If recent contact information for these individuals cannot be obtained, more public notice via the covered entity's website or through media publications may be required. P.L. 111-5, § 13402(e)(1)(B).
[66] The list is at http://www.hhs.gov/ocr/privacy/hipaa/administrative/breachnotificationrule/postedbreaches.html.

[67] P.L. 111-5, § 13402(i). The first such report was due February 17, 2010. *Id.*
[68] 74 Fed. Reg. 42740 (August 24, 2009). *See also* 45 C.F.R. §§ 164.400 *et seq.*
[69] P.L. 111-5, § 13407(g)(2). For further information on electronic personal health records, *see* CRS Report RS22760, *Electronic Personal Health Records*, by Gina Stevens.
[70] The FTC is directed to also notify the Secretary of HHS in the event of a breach.
[71] P.L. 111-5, § 13407(f)(1).
[72] P.L. 111-5, § 13407(f)(2).
[73] *See* CRS Report RL34120, *Federal Information Security and Data Breach Notification Laws*, by Gina Stevens, at 16-17.
[74] 16 C.F.R. part. 318.
[75] P.L. 111-5, § 13403(a). On July 27, 2009, the Secretary, through the OCR, designated the OCR Regional Managers as Regional Office Privacy Officers. *See* http://www.hhs.gov/ocr/privacy/hipaa/understanding/coveredentities/ ropadesignation.html.
[76] P.L. 111-5, § 13403(b).
[77] P.L. 111-5, § 13404(a).
[78] P.L. 111-5, § 13404(a).
[79] 45 C.F.R. § 164.504(e)(1)(ii).
[80] P.L. 111-5, § 13404(b).
[81] P.L. 111-5, §§ 13401(b), 13404(c).
[82] 45 C.F.R. § 164.502(b)(1). The minimum necessary standard does not apply to disclosures that are authorized by an individual, are made for the treatment of the individual, or are made directly to the individual. Disclosures that were required by law or other provisions of the HIPAA Privacy Rule, or are made to the Secretary for compliance or investigatory purposes, are also not subject to the minimum necessary standard.
[83] 45 C.F.R. § 164.514(e)(3).
[84] 45 C.F.R. § 164.514(e)(2).
[85] P.L. 111-5, § 13405(b)(1)(A).
[86] P.L. 111-5, § 13405(b)(1)(B). The deadline for this guidance was February 17, 2010.
[87] P.L. 111-5, § 13405(b)(1)(C).
[88] P.L. 111-5, § 13405(b)(2).
[89] 45 C.F.R. § 164.528(a)(1)(i).
[90] P.L. 111-5, § 13405(c)(4).
[91] 45 C.F.R. § 164.508(a)(3)(ii).
[92] P.L. 111-5, § 13405(d).
[93] P.L. 111-5, § 13405(d)(2)(B).
[94] P.L. 111-5, § 13405(d)(2)(C).
[95] P.L. 111-5, § 13405(d)(2)(F).
[96] P.L. 111-5, § 13405(d)(2)(A).
[97] P.L. 111-5, § 13405(d)(3)(A).
[98] P.L. 111-5, § 13405(d)(3)(B).
[99] P.L. 111-5, § 13405(d)(2)(E).
[100] P.L. 111-5, § 13405(d)(2)(D).
[101] P.L. 111-5, § 13405(d)(2)(G).
[102] P.L. 111-5, § 13405(d)(4). The Secretary is also directed to issue regulations to carry out this subsection by August 17, 2010. P.L. 111-5, § 13405(d)(3).
[103] P.L. 111-5, § 13405(e)(2).
[104] P.L. 111-5, § 13406(c).
[105] 45 C.F.R. § 164.501.
[100] P.L. 111-5, § 13405(d)(2)(D).
[101] P.L. 111-5, § 13405(d)(2)(G).
[102] P.L. 111-5, § 13405(d)(4). The Secretary is also directed to issue regulations to carry out this subsection by August 17, 2010. P.L. 111-5, § 13405(d)(3).
[103] P.L. 111-5, § 13405(e)(2).
[104] P.L. 111-5, § 13406(c).
[105] 45 C.F.R. § 164.501.
[106] *Id.*
[107] 45 C.F.R. § 164.508(a)(3)(i).

[108] P.L. 111-5, § 13406(a)(1). *See also* H.Rept. 111-16, at 497-8.
[109] P.L. 111-5, § 13406(a)(2).
[110] P.L. 111-5, § 13406(a)(2)(A).
[111] P.L. 111-5, § 13406(a)(2)(A)(ii).
[112] P.L. 111-5, § 13406(a)(3).
[113] P.L. 111-5, § 13406(a)(2)(C).
[114] 45 C.F.R. § 164.506(a).
[115] 45 C.F.R. § 164.501.
[116] 45 C.F.R. § 164.520(b)(1)(iii)(B).
[117] 45 C.F.R. § 164.514(f)(1).
[118] 45 C.F.R. § 164.514(f)(2).
[119] H.Rept. 111-16, at 498.
[120] *Id.* at 497.
[121] P.L. 111-5, § 13408.
[122] *Id.*
[123] P.L. 111-5, § 13409.
[124] CRS Report RL33989, *Enforcement of the HIPAA Privacy and Security Rules*, by Gina Stevens.
[125] P.L. 111-5, § 13410(b)(1).
[126] 42 U.S.C. § 1320d-5(b)(1).
[127] P.L. 111-5, § 13410(a)(1)(A).
[128] P.L. 111-5, § 13410(a)(1)(B).
[129] 42 U.S.C. § 1320d-5(a)(1)(A-C).
[130] 42 U.S.C. § 1320d-5(d)(1)(A).
[131] 42 U.S.C. § 1320d-5(b)(2)(A).
[132] 42 U.S.C. § 1320d-5(a)(1)(B).
[133] 42 U.S.C. § 1320d-5(b)(2)(A).
[134] 42 U.S.C. § 1320d-5(a)(1)(C)(i).
[135] 42 U.S.C. § 1320d-5(a)(1)(C)(ii)
[136] *See Acara v. Banks*, 470 F.3d 569 (finding no explicit or implicit private cause of action under HIPAA).
[137] P.L. 111-5, § 13410(e)(3).
[138] 42 U.S.C. § 1320d-5(d)(8).
[139] 42 U.S.C. § 1320d-5(d)(4).
[140] 42 U.S.C. § 1320d-5(d)(7).
[141] 42 U.S.C. § 1320d-5(d)(3).
[142] *Gulf Offshore Co. v. Mobil Oil Corp.*, 453 U.S. 473 (1981).
[143] P.L. 111-5, § 13410(e)(1) (emphasis added).
[144] *Tafflin v. Levitt*, 493 U.S. 455, 460 (1990) (emphasis added). *See also Yellow Freight Sys. Inc. v. Donnelly*, 494 U.S. 820, 840 (1990) (the omission of a provision in Title VII of the Civil Rights Act of 1964 expressly limiting the presumed concurrent jurisdiction of state courts is strong, and arguably sufficient, evidence that Congress had no such intent).
[145] H.Rept. 111-16, at 501.
[146] H.Rept. 111-7, to accompany H.R. 629 ("this provision authorizes state attorneys general to enforce federal privacy and security laws"); H.Rept. 111-8, to accompany H.R. 598 ("the bill would authorize state Attorneys General to bring a civil action in federal district court against individuals who violate the HIPAA privacy and security standards"); S.Rept. 111-3, to accompany S. 336 (without additional commentary on provision).
[147] During the markup of H.R. 629, an amendment was offered by Rep. Rogers to strike the entire section authorizing state attorneys general to pursue civil enforcement, but was not agreed to. The debate over that amendment did not include any discussion of whether federal courts should enjoy exclusive jurisdiction over such claims.
[148] *Gulf Offshore Co. v. Mobil Oil Corp.*, 453 U.S. at 483-484.
[149] *Tafflin, supra* note 11.
[150] *Yellow Freight Sys., supra* note 11.
[151] *Charles Dowd Box Co. v. Courtney*, 368 U.S. 502 (1962).
[152] 28 U.S.C. § 1441.

[153] OFFICE OF THE ATTORNEY GENERAL OF CONNECTICUT, *Press Release: Attorney General Sues Health Net For Massive Security Breach Involving Private Medical Records And Financial Information On 446,000 Enrollees*, January 13, 2010.
[154] P.L. 111-5, § 13411.
[155] P.L. 111-5, § 13421(a).
[156] P.L. 111-5, § 13421(b).
[157] *Id.*
[158] P.L. 111-5, § 13424(a).
[159] P.L. 111-5, § 13424(a)(1).
[160] P.L. 111-5, § 13424(b). The deadline for this study was February 17, 2010.
[161] P.L. 111-5, § 13424(c).
[162] P.L. 111-5, § 13424(f).
[163] P.L. 111-5, § 13424(d). The deadline for this report was February 17, 2010.
[164] P.L. 111-5, § 13424(e).

In: Transforming Healthcare with Health Information… ISBN: 978-1-61324-417-3
Editors: C. M. Denison, E. L. Montevoy

Chapter 4

Nationwide Privacy and Security Framework for Electronic Exchange of Individually Identifiable Health Information*

Office of the National Coordinator for Health Information Technology

I. Preamble to the Nationwide Privacy and Security Framework for Electronic Exchange of Individually Identifiable Health Information

Purpose

Electronic health information exchange promises an array of potential benefits for individuals and the U.S. health care system through improved clinical care and reduced cost. At the same time, this environment also poses new challenges and opportunities for protecting individually identifiable health information. In health care, accurate and complete information about individuals is critical to providing high quality, coordinated care. If individuals and other participants in a network lack trust in electronic exchange of information due to perceived or actual risks to individually identifiable health information or the accuracy and completeness of such information, it may affect their willingness to disclose necessary health information and could have life-threatening consequences. A key factor to achieving a high level of trust among individuals, health care providers, and other health care organizations participating in electronic health information exchange is the development of, and adherence to, a consistent and coordinated approach to privacy and security. Clear, understandable, uniform principles are a first step in developing a consistent and coordinated approach to privacy and security and a key component to building the trust required to realize the potential benefits of electronic health information exchange.

---

* This is an edited, reformatted and augmented version of the U.S. Department of Health and Human Services publication, dated December 15, 2008.

The principles below establish a single, consistent approach to address the privacy and security challenges related to electronic health information exchange through a network for all persons, regardless of the legal framework that may apply to a particular organization. The goal of this effort is to establish a policy framework for electronic health information exchange that can help guide the Nation's adoption of health information technologies and help improve the availability of health information and health care quality. The principles have been designed to establish the roles of individuals and the responsibilities of those who hold and exchange electronic individually identifiable health information through a network.

Background

Numerous forces are driving the health care industry towards the use of health information technology, such as the potential for reducing medical errors and health care costs, and increasing individuals' involvement in their own health and health care. To facilitate this advancement and reap its benefits while reducing the risks, it is important to consider individual privacy interests together with the potential benefits to population health.

Historical Perspective

The Federal government has long recognized the importance of privacy and security protections for the electronic collection, use, and disclosure of individually identifiable information and principles or practices to guide those actions. As early as 1973, the U.S. Department of Health, Education, and Welfare (HEW) appointed the Advisory Committee on Automated Personal Data Systems to analyze the consequences of using computers to keep records about people. In order to benefit from computerization while providing privacy safeguards, the advisory committee developed the *Code of Fair Information Practice*, which addresses five practices: openness, disclosure, secondary use, correction, and security. These practices have influenced many U.S. laws at both the Federal and state levels and also numerous other national and international documents. For example, in 1974, the Privacy Act was passed, which protects certain personal information held by Federal agencies. In 1980, the Organisation for Economic Cooperation and Development (OECD), an international organization comprised of 24 countries including the U.S., published a consensus document, the *Guidelines on the Protection of Privacy and Transborder Flows of Personal Data*. The purpose of the Guidelines was to decrease disparities and assist in harmonizing legislation that would allow the flow of data while preventing violations of what the OECD member countries considered fundamental human rights. In 1998, the Federal Trade Commission published *Privacy Online: a Report to Congress,* which among other conclusions stated that effective self-regulation is the preferred approach to protecting individuals' privacy. Most recently, the U.S. Department of Health and Human Services (HHS) built on these principles in developing the Privacy Rule under the Health Insurance Portability and Accountability Act of 1996 (HIPAA).

In 2004, the Office of the National Coordinator for Health Information Technology (ONC) was created by E.O. 13335, which charged the National Coordinator to the extent permitted by law, to develop, maintain, and direct the implementation of, a strategic plan to guide the nationwide implementation of interoperable health information technology in both the public and private health care sectors and to address in the plan, among other things, "privacy and security issues related to interoperable health information technology and recommend methods to ensure appropriate authorization, authentication, and encryption of data for transmission over the Internet…"

Legal Environment

Over several decades, states have passed laws to protect the privacy of health information. These laws differ from state to state and often narrowly target a particular population, health condition, data collection effort, or specific types of health care organizations. As a result, states have created a patchwork of privacy protections that are not comprehensive or easily understood. Many states also have begun to consider information security related issues and have passed laws, for example, requiring various types of entities to provide notice of security breaches of individually identifiable information.

At the Federal level, there are also a variety of laws related to the privacy and security of health information, including the HIPAA Privacy and Security Rules, the Privacy Act of 1974, the Confidentiality of Alcohol and Drug Abuse Patient Records Regulation (42 CFR Part 2), the Family Educational Rights & Privacy Act (addresses privacy of information held by certain educational institutions), Gramm-Leach-Bliley Financial

Services Act (addresses privacy of information held by financial institutions), and Federal Information Security Management Act of 2002 (FISMA).

The Privacy and Security Rules promulgated under HIPAA were the first Federal regulations to broadly address the privacy and security of health information. They establish a baseline of national privacy and security standards for individually identifiable health information held by "covered entities" and a foundation of protection regardless of health condition, type of health program, population, state where the activity occurs, or other situational characteristics.

Although the HIPAA Privacy and Security Rules apply to health information in electronic form, the current landscape of electronic health information exchange poses new issues and involves additional organizations that were not contemplated at the time the rules were drafted.

Methodology

In the development of the Nationwide Privacy and Security Framework for Electronic Exchange of Individually Identifiable Health Information, ONC reviewed various international, national, and public and private sector privacy and security principles that focused on individual information in an electronic environment (but not necessarily on health), including those that focused on individually identifiable health information. This review included:

- HEW Advisory Committee's Code of Fair Information Practice[i]
- Markle Foundation's Connecting Consumers: Common Framework for Networked Personal Health Information[ii]
- Organisation for Economic Co-operation and Development (OECD) Guidelines on the Protection of Privacy and Transborder Flows of Personal Data[iii]
- Health Information Technology – Consumer Principles[iv]

- Federal Trade Commission's Privacy Online: A Report to Congress – Fair Information Practice Principles[v]
- The International Security Trust and Privacy Alliance's (ISTPA): Privacy Framework[vi]

It is worth noting that ISTPA conducted a privacy and security principles analysis and harmonization, while accommodating variation from the following instruments, which resulted in the ISTPA principles reviewed by HHS:

- The Privacy Act of 1974
- OECD Guidelines on the Protection of Privacy and Transborder Flows of Personal Data
- UN Guidelines Concerning Personalized Computer Files
- EU Data Protection Directive 95/46/EC
- Canadian Standards Association Model Code (incorporated in the Personal Information Protection and Electronic Documents Act [PIPEDA])
- Health Insurance Portability and Accountability Act of 1996 (HIPAA) Privacy Rules
- US FTC Statement of Fair Information Practice Principles
- US-EU Safe Harbor Privacy Principles
- Australian Privacy Act – National Privacy Principles
- Japan Personal Information Protection Act
- APEC (Asia-Pacific Economic Cooperation) Privacy Framework

There was a great deal of commonality across these principles. After a careful review and analysis of these principles, we harmonized them while accommodating as much variation as possible and being careful to consider how they may apply to electronic health information exchange. We also reviewed the approaches taken by various Federal laws, specifically the HIPAA Privacy and Security Rules, the Privacy Act, and FISMA, as well as recommendations that the Secretary had approved from two advisory committees, the National Committee on Vital and Health Statistics (NCVHS) and the American Health Information Community (AHIC).

Principles

The principles outlined in the Nationwide Privacy and Security Framework for Electronic Exchange of Individually Identifiable Health Information serve as a guide for public and private-sector entities that hold or exchange electronic individually identifiable health information and the development of any compliance and enforcement approaches, including industry self-regulation. Additionally, these principles are designed to complement and work with existing Federal, state, territorial, local, and tribal laws and regulations and should not be construed or interpreted as supplanting or altering any applicable laws or regulations. Various Federal Government agencies are expected to look to these principles as the framework for their policy and technology activities in this area and to encourage states and private sector organizations to do the same.

The implementation of these principles should be dynamic and subject to modification as information practices and technologies advance; however, these principles are designed to be applicable as technology changes.

Scope

These principles are expected to guide the actions of all health care-related persons and entities that participate in a network for the purpose of electronic exchange of individually identifiable health information. These principles are not intended to apply to individuals with respect to their own individually identifiable health information.

By adopting these principles, persons and entities will follow a common approach to privacy and security and develop appropriate and comparable protections for information, thereby increasing trust in electronic exchange of individually identifiable health information. These principles do not apply to individuals with respect to their own individually identifiable health information. Individuals may use and/or disclose their individual health information as they choose. For example, an individual may share details of a chronic disease on the Internet or in a public meeting but may decide not to share that information with all his or her health care providers or employers. Likewise, an individual should not be expected to implement the administrative responsibilities of these principles such as developing policies and procedures.

Organization of the Principles

The framework is comprised eight principles that are organized as follows:

- Principles (Level I): Each principle is made up of a short title and a concise statement designed to clearly and simply reflect the concept embodied within each: Individual Access; Correction; Openness and Transparency; Individual Choice; Collection, Use, and Disclosure Limitation; Data Quality and Integrity; Safeguards; and Accountability.
- Detail (Level II): Each principle is followed by a short explanation that further elaborates on the principle, what it is designed to do, and its parameters.

Terminology

In order to best understand the scope and application of the principles, it is recommended that the reader refer to the glossary (Appendix 1), particularly with respect to the definitions of "individuals" and "persons and entities."

II. The Nationwide Privacy and Security Framework for Electronic Exchange of Individually Identifiable Health Information

Scope

These principles are expected to guide the actions of all health care-related persons and entities that participate in a network for the purpose of electronic exchange of individually identifiable health information. These principles are not intended to apply to individuals with respect to their own individually identifiable health information.

Introduction

Adoption of privacy and security protections is essential to establishing the public trust necessary for effective electronic exchange of individually identifiable health information. A common set of principles that stakeholders accept and support is the first step towards realizing those privacy and security protections and establishing the necessary public trust. The approach of developing principles to guide information practices while advancing technology was marked by the 1973 release of the Code of Fair Information Practice and has been the basis for various activities in the public and private sectors, including the development of the Health Insurance Portability and Accountability Act (HIPAA) Privacy Rule and as the basis for this framework.

The implementation of these principles should evolve in concert with technological advances that allow for greater protections. Adherence should be the responsibility of each health care-related person or entity that holds and exchanges electronic individually identifiable health information through a network, as well as the responsibility of other persons and entities that receive or have access to such information, so that electronic individually identifiable health information is protected at all times.

These principles do not constitute legal advice and do not affect a person's or entity's duty to comply with applicable legal requirements. Where these principles set higher standards than legal requirements, adherence to these principles is encouraged.

Individual Access

Individuals should be provided with a simple and timely means to access and obtain their individually identifiable health information in a readable form and format.

Access to information enables individuals to manage their health care and well-being. Individuals should have a reasonable means of access to their individually identifiable health information. Individuals should be able to obtain this information easily, consistent with security needs for authentication of the individual; and such information should be provided promptly so as to be useful for managing their health. Additionally, the persons and entities, that participate in a network for the purpose of electronic exchange of individually identifiable health information, should provide such information in a readable form and format, including an electronic format, when appropriate. In limited instances, medical or other circumstances may result in the appropriate denial of individual access to their health information.

Correction

Individuals should be provided with a timely means to dispute the accuracy or integrity of their individually identifiable health information, and to have erroneous information corrected or to have a dispute documented if their requests are denied.

Individuals have an important stake in the accuracy and integrity of their individually identifiable health information and an important role to play in ensuring its accuracy and integrity. Electronic exchange of individually identifiable health information may improve care and reduce adverse events. However, any errors or conclusions drawn from erroneous data may be easily communicated or replicated (e.g., as a result of an administrative error as simple as a transposed digit or more complex error arising from medical identity theft). For this reason it is essential for individuals to have practical, efficient, and timely means for disputing the accuracy or integrity of their individually identifiable health information, to have this information corrected, or a dispute documented when their requests are denied, and to have the correction or dispute communicated to others with whom the underlying information has been shared. Persons and entities, that participate in a network for the purpose of electronic exchange of individually identifiable health information, should make processes available to empower individuals to exercise a role in managing their individually identifiable health information and should correct information or document disputes in a timely fashion.

Openness and Transparency

There should be openness and transparency about policies, procedures, and technologies that directly affect individuals and/or their individually identifiable health information.

Trust in electronic exchange of individually identifiable health information can best be established in an open and transparent environment. Individuals should be able to understand what individually identifiable health information exists about them, how that individually identifiable health information is collected, used, and disclosed and whether and how they can exercise choice over such collections, uses, and disclosures. Persons and entities, that participate in a network for the purpose of electronic exchange of individually identifiable health information, should provide reasonable opportunities for individuals to review who has accessed their individually identifiable health information or to whom it has been disclosed, in a readable form and format. Notice of policies, procedures, and technology-- including what information will be provided under what circumstances -- should be timely and, wherever possible, made in advanced of the collection, use, and/or disclosure of individually identifiable he

information. Policies and procedures developed consistent with this Nationwide Privacy and Security Framework for Electronic Exchange of Individually Identifiable Health

Information should be communicated in a manner that is appropriate and understandable to individuals.

Individual Choice

Individuals should be provided a reasonable opportunity and capability to make informed decisions about the collection, use, and disclosure of their individually identifiable health information.

The ability of individuals to make choices with respect to electronic exchange of individually identifiable health information concerning them is important to building trust. Persons and entities, that participate in a network for the purpose of electronic exchange of individually identifiable health information, should provide reasonable opportunities and capabilities for individuals to exercise choice with respect to their individually identifiable health information. The degree of choice made available may vary with the type of information being exchanged, the purpose of the exchange, and the recipient of the information. Applicable law, population health needs, medical necessity, ethical principles, and technology, among other factors, may affect options for expressing choice. Individuals should be able to designate someone else, such as a family member, care-giver, or legal guardian, to make decisions on their behalf. When an individual exercises choice, including the ability to designate someone else to make decisions on his or her behalf, the process should be fair and not unduly burdensome.

Collection, Use, and Disclosure Limitation

Individually identifiable health information should be collected, used, and/or disclosed only to the extent necessary to accomplish a specified purpose(s) and never to discriminate inappropriately.

Establishing appropriate limits on the type and amount of information collected, used, and/or disclosed increases privacy protections and is essential to building trust in electronic exchange of individually identifiable health information because it minimizes potential misuse and abuse. Persons and entities, that participate in a network for the purpose of electronic exchange *of individually identifiable health information, should only collect, use, and/or disclose information necessary to accomplish a specified purpose(s). Persons and entities should take advantage of technological advances to limit data collection, use, and/or disclosure.*

Data Quality and Integrity

Persons and entities should take reasonable steps to ensure that individually identifiable health information is complete, accurate, and up-to-date to the extent necessary for the person's or entity's intended purposes and has not been altered or destroyed in an unauthorized manner.

The completeness and accuracy of an individual's health information may affect, among other things, the quality of care that the individual receives, medical decisions, and health outcomes. Persons and entities, that participate in a network for the purpose of electronic exchange of individually identifiable health information, have a responsibility to maintain individually identifiable health information that is useful for its intended purposes, which involves taking reasonable steps to ensure that information is accurate, complete, and up-to-date, and has not been altered or destroyed in an unauthorized manner. Persons and entities have a responsibility to update or correct individually identifiable health information and to provide timely notice of these changes to others with whom the underlying information has been shared. Moreover, persons and entities should develop processes to detect, prevent, and mitigate any unauthorized changes to, or deletions of, individually identifiable health information.

Safeguards

Individually identifiable health information should be protected with reasonable administrative, technical, and physical safeguards to ensure its confidentiality, integrity, and availability and to prevent unauthorized or inappropriate access, use, or disclosure.

Trust in electronic exchange of individually identifiable health information can only be achieved if reasonable administrative, technical, and physical safeguards are in place to protect individually identifiable health information and minimize the risks of unauthorized or inappropriate access, use, or disclosure. These safeguards should be developed after a thorough assessment to determine any risks or vulnerabilities to individually identifiable health information. Persons and entities, that participate in a network for the purpose of electronic exchange of individually identifiable health information, should implement administrative, technical, and physical safeguards to protect information, including assuring that only authorized persons and entities and employees of such persons or entities have access to individually identifiable health information. Administrative, technical, and physical safeguards should be reasonable in scope and balanced with the need for access to individually identifiable health information.

Accountability

These principles should be implemented, and adherence assured, through appropriate monitoring and other means and methods should be in place to report and mitigate non-adherence and breaches.

These nationwide privacy and security principles will not be effective in building trust in electronic exchange of individually identifiable health information unless there is compliance with these Principles and enforcement mechanisms. Mechanisms for assuring accountability include policies and procedures and other tools. At a minimum, such mechanisms adopted by persons and entities, that participate in a network for the purpose of electronic exchange of individually identifiable health information, should address: (1) monitoring for internal compliance including authentication and authorizations for access to or disclosure of individually identifiable health information; (2) the ability to receive and act on complaints, including taking corrective measures; and (3) the provision of reasonable mitigation measures, including notice to individuals of privacy violations or security breaches that pose substantial risk of harm to such individuals.

End Notes

[i] The U.S. Department of Health, Education and Welfare now the U.S. Department of Health and Human Services: http://www.hhs.gov/*Report of the Secretary's Advisory Committee on Automated Personal Data Systems* (1973): http://aspe.hhs.gov/DATACNCL/1973privacy/tocprefacemembers.htm

[ii] Markle Foundation: http://www.markle.org/*Common Framework for Networked Personal Health Information: Overview and Principles (Current as of 2008):* http://www.connectingforhealth.org/phti/reports/overview.html

[iii] Organisation for Economic Co-operation and Development (OECD): *http://www.oecd.org/home/0,2987,en_2649_201185_1_1_1_1_1,00.html Guidelines on the Protection of Privacy and Transborder Flows of Personal Data (1980): http://www.oecd.org/document/18/0,3343,en_2649_34255_1815186_1_1_1_1,00.html*

[iv] *Health Information Technology – Consumer Principles* (2006), Endorsed by: AARP AFL-CIO; American Federation of State, County and Municipal Employees; American Federation of Teachers; Center for Medical Consumers; Communications Workers of America; Consumers Union; Department for Professional Employees, AFL-CIO; Childbirth Connection Health Care for All; Health Privacy Project; International Association of Machinists and Aerospace Workers; International Union, United Auto Workers; National Coalition for Cancer Survivorship; National Consumers League; National Partnership for Women & Families; Service Employees International Union; Title II Community AIDS National Network; United Steelworkers International Union (USW): http://www.nclnet.org/health/final%202006%20principles%20PDF.pdf

[v] Federal Trade Commission (FTC): http://www.ftc.gov/Privacy Online: A Report to Congress (1998) – Fair Information Practice Principles: http://www.ftc.gov/reports/privacy3/fairinfo.shtm

[vi] International Security Trust and Privacy Alliance (ISTPA): www.istpa.org Analysis of Privacy Principles: An Operational Study (2007, Version 1.8): http://www.istpa.org/pdfs/ISTPAAnalysisofPrivacyPrinciplesV2.pdf

APPENDIX I: GLOSSARY

Administrative safeguards: Administrative actions, and policies and procedures to manage the selection, development, implementation, and maintenance of security measures to protect electronic individually identifiable health information and to manage the conduct of the entity's workforce in relation to the protection of that information. Administrative safeguards include policies and procedures, workforce training, risk management plans, and contingency plans.

Collect/Collection: The acquisition or receipt of information, including individually identifiable health information.

Corrective measures: Actions taken to address a security breach or privacy violation, with the intent to counteract the breach or violation and reduce future risks.

Disclose/Disclosure: The release, transfer, exchange, provision of access to, or divulging in any other manner of information outside the person or entity holding the information.

Health Information: Any information that relates to the past, present, or future physical or mental health or condition of an individual; the provision of health care to an individual; or the past, present, or future payment for the provision of health care to an individual.

Individual: A person who is the recipient of health and/or wellness services.

Individually Identifiable Health Information: Health information that identifies the individual, or with respect to which there is a reasonable basis to believe the information can be used to identify the individual.

Open: Actively communicating information through notice or otherwise.

Persons and Entities: Health care professionals, partnerships, proprietorships, corporations and other types of organizations and their agents when acting on their behalf.

Physical safeguards: Physical measures, policies and procedures to protect electronic information systems and related buildings and equipment from natural and environmental hazards, and unauthorized intrusion. Physical safeguards include workstation security and use procedures, facility security plans, data backup and storage, and portable device and media controls.

Privacy: An individual's interest in protecting his or her individually identifiable health information and the corresponding obligation of those persons and entities, that participate in a network for the purposes of electronic exchange of such information, to respect those interests through fair information practices.

Security: The physical, technological, and administrative safeguards used to protect individually identifiable health information.

Technical safeguards: The technology and the policies and procedures for its use that protect electronic individually identifiable health information and control access to it.

Transparent: Making information readily and publicly available.

Use: Is the employment, application, utilization, examination, analysis or maintenance of individually identifiable health information.

INDEX

A

B

C

G

H

N

O

P

Q

R

S

T

U

V

W

X

Y